Nurses' Aids Series
SPECIAL INTEREST TEXTS

OPHTHALMIC NURSING

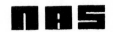

NURSES' AIDS SERIES

ANATOMY AND PHYSIOLOGY FOR NURSES
EAR, NOSE AND THROAT NURSING
GERIATRIC NURSING
MATHEMATICS IN NURSING
MEDICAL NURSING
MICROBIOLOGY FOR NURSES
MULTIPLE CHOICE QUESTIONS, BOOK 1
MULTIPLE CHOICE QUESTIONS, BOOK 2
MULTIPLE CHOICE QUESTIONS, BOOK 3
OBSTETRIC AND GYNAECOLOGICAL NURSING
PAEDIATRIC NURSING
PERSONAL AND COMMUNITY HEALTH
PHARMACOLOGY FOR NURSES
PRACTICAL NURSING
PRACTICAL PROCEDURES FOR NURSES
PSYCHIATRIC NURSING
PSYCHOLOGY FOR NURSES
SOCIOLOGY FOR NURSES
SURGICAL NURSING
THEATRE TECHNIQUE

SPECIAL INTEREST TEXTS

ACCIDENT AND EMERGENCY NURSING
ANAESTHESIA AND RECOVERY ROOM TECHNIQUES
GASTROENTEROLOGICAL NURSING
NEUROMEDICAL AND NEUROSURGICAL NURSING
NUTRITION AND DIETETICS IN HEALTH AND DISEASE
OPHTHALMIC NURSING
ORTHOPAEDICS FOR NURSES

Nurses' Aids Series
SPECIAL INTEREST TEXTS

Ophthalmic Nursing

Second Edition

Vera H. Darling
OND, SRN, BTA Cert, RNT
Principal Officer, Joint Board
of Clinical Nursing Studies

and

Margaret R. Thorpe
OND, SRN, Diploma in Nursing (Lond), RNT
Health Education Officer,
Croydon Area Health Authority

BAILLIÈRE TINDALL · LONDON

A BAILLIÈRE TINDALL book published by
Cassell Ltd.
35 Red Lion Square, London WC1R 4SG

and at Sydney, Auckland, Toronto, Johannesburg

an affiliate of
Macmillan Publishing Co. Inc.
New York

First published 1975
   Reprinted 1979
Second edition 1981

ISBN 0 7020 0829 X

Printed in Great Britain by Lowe & Brydone (Printers) Ltd, Thetford, Norfolk

British Library Cataloguing in Publication Data

Darling, Vera Hannah
   Ophthalmic nursing. — 2nd ed. — (Nurses' aids
   series: special interest texts).
   1. Ophthalmic nursing   2. Eyes — Diseases
   and defects
   I. Title   II. Series
   617.7'002'4613   RE88
   ISBN 0-7020-0829-X

Contents

	List of Colour Plates	vi
	Preface	vii
1	Ophthalmic Nurse and Patient	1
2	Caring for Ophthalmic Patients	4
3	Eye Drops and Medications	27
4	The Lens	33
5	The Retina	61
6	The Vitreous and Aqueous Humour	78
7	The Uveal Tract	96
8	The Cornea and Sclera	104
9	The Conjunctiva	118
10	The Lacrimal Apparatus	127
11	The Extraocular Muscles	133
12	The Protective Structures	140
13	Ophthalmic Conditions of Tropical Climates	157
14	Enucleation	167
15	Blindness	172
	Glossary	177
	Index	182

Colour Plates

between pages 88 *and* 89

PLATE I The fundus

1   The normal fundus
2   Occlusion of the central retinal artery
3   Thrombosis of a branch retinal vein

PLATE II The 'red eye'

1   Acute closed angle glaucoma
2   Acute follicular conjunctivitis
3   Iridocyclitis

Preface

Ophthalmic nursing requires a special combination of skill and understanding. This book has been written primarily for the nurse who, in the course of general training, is on the threshold of gaining that combination in the ophthalmic ward, clinic or unit. However those undergoing specialized training in ophthalmic nursing will also find this second edition a useful concise text.

In this edition the chapter on Caring for Ophthalmic Patients has been rearranged to bring it in line with the current thinking on the models of patient care and replaces the chapter on Procedures and Techniques. With the increasing use of contact lenses and the recent developments in the use of lasers and phako-emulsification, the sections on these topics have been expanded. The chapter on Blindness has been completely rewritten to take account of the advances in care and the facilities available for the visually handicapped.

In the United Kingdom and other countries in temperate climates, the ophthalmic nurse will commonly encounter such conditions as cataract, glaucoma, infections and retinal separation; in industrial areas, eye injuries will also be frequently seen.

In certain tropical areas of the world, not only will these conditions be met but the nurse will see patients suffering from trachoma, onchocerciasis and ophthalmia neonatorum together with ophthalmic conditions resulting from malnutrition. A chapter on tropical diseases has been included.

The chapters have been arranged in order to integrate topics related to particular conditions of the eye. We felt that this would give the nurse the necessary knowledge to assess the needs of the patient, to plan the nursing care required by the patient and to establish an awareness of the follow-up care of each patient she looks after.

In preparing the second edition we would particularly like to thank the following people who have given so generously of their time. Miss Sinlan Lim, Mr Brian Patton and Miss Marion Worsel. Our thanks are also due to the staff of Baillière Tindall for their considerable advice and encouragement.

We are also grateful to the following for supplying illustrations for inclusion in the book: Clement Clarke International Ltd for Figs 13 and 31; Croydon Eye Unit for Fig. 16; Dr D.W. Ellis-Jones for Fig. 55; Mr David Fletcher for Fig. 18; Mr G. Green and the Department of Photography, Princess Margaret Hospital, Swindon, for Figs 19, 20, 21 and 22; Hamblin (Instruments) Ltd for Figs 25 and 34; Keeler Instruments Ltd for Fig. 17; Mr F.D. Rodger and the Department of Photography, Princess Margaret Hospital, Swindon, for Figs 6, 7, 26, 30, 40, 41, 45, 54 and 57; and Dr Phillip Rodin, The London Hospital, for Fig. 39.

VERA H. DARLING
MARGARET R. THORPE

September 1980

1

Ophthalmic Nurse and Patient

The student nurse in her training will have had experience in more general nursing before she enters the specialized field of the ophthalmic ward, out-patient department or perhaps operating theatre. However, wherever she has the care of a patient with an ophthalmic condition, whether caused by disease or injury, it is important for her to realize that the patient will need a special kind of skill and understanding. She has only to try to imagine what it would mean to herself to lose what many people may feel to be the most precious of the senses to appreciate the fear that many patients, admitted to an ophthalmic ward or hospital, may have of loss of vision.

Some patients will already have suffered impaired vision for some time, for example those with cataracts, particularly when the condition is bilateral; others may have normal sight which is jeopardized by sudden, serious injury, perhaps in a traffic accident or as a result of carelessly handled fireworks.

The patient with a long-standing condition will in all probability already have adjusted to his impairment of vision, whatever the degree, but on admission to hospital will need sympathetic handling in accustoming himself to new surroundings and strange people so that his confidence is built up to withstand his fear that perhaps treatment may not be successful. In the case of sudden injury, where the nursing care will include the treatment of shock, it is even more important for the nurse to realize the fear and apprehension that the patient will inevitably experience. He may be in considerable pain, bewildered, confused and frightened.

The nurse used to a busy general surgical or medical ward often finds the ophthalmic ward or hospital very quiet. There are seldom any dramatic emergencies and she may have to adapt her approach and general tempo of work in order that the quieter and slower pace of the ophthalmic patient is not disturbed. When she understands this she will be able to use the skills she has already acquired in dealing with the sick to help those who are suffering from impaired vision and who may be very apprehensive of what the future holds for them. The nurse should use every opportunity that arises to talk to the patient and help him to cope with his disability, both physically and psychologically.

Although the patients all have disorders of one small special organ, a number of them may have other conditions which may or may not be a contributory factor to the eye condition that has brought them to hospital, and the nurse should watch carefully for any signs of general organic disease. In doing so she will develop her skills of observation and reporting on the patients in her care. The nurse will have to consider how patients with limited vision can appreciate the other special senses and help them to make the best use of them.

The ophthalmic nurse must be gentle and dextrous in using her hands when carrying out procedures. Before undertaking any treatment she will explain what she is about to do to the patient in order to gain his confidence and cooperation. When approaching a patient who is unable to see, the nurse should speak quietly to him by name in order to make her presence known, and when walking with him should allow him to hold her lightly by the arm if he is unfamiliar with his surroundings. Never should the patient be pushed along from behind. The nurse should tell the patient when she is about to leave him and see that he is comfortable with all the things he may need to hand, their position known.

Nursing of ophthalmic patients can be very rewarding, especially in terms of the help and sympathetic support that the nurse can give to her patient in these circumstances. If there is a possibility of the patient becoming blind there is an even greater need for support by the nurse. She can help by letting the patient talk out his fears and by so doing begin to face a future without sight. The nurse should have some knowledge of what practical steps can be taken to help blind people to lead a life as nearly normal as possible and this subject is dealt with in the chapter on blindness.

For those whose vision can be improved by treatment and operative procedures the nurse will have the satisfaction of knowing that she has contributed to a return to a fuller life by the patient.

2

Caring for Ophthalmic Patients

THE ADULT PATIENT

PREOPERATIVE CARE

When possible the patient is admitted to the ward 24 hours before operation. This not only gives him time to adapt to the new situation and routine, but also enables the nursing staff to interview him in order to formulate the nursing care plan and give him a careful explanation of the pre- and postoperative measures to be carried out, thus gaining his confidence and cooperation and reinforcing the explanation given to him by the surgeon in the out-patient department when he may have been too agitated to understand completely. The patient is welcomed to the ward and personal details and habits, such as sleeping and eating, are recorded.

He is then taken round the ward, introduced to the other patients and shown where the bathroom and toilets are. It must be remembered that patients may have very poor sight and feel confused and insecure in unfamiliar surroundings, so that great care should be taken over helping them to settle in and gain a sense of belonging. The attitude of the nurse who first greets the patient is of the utmost importance; if his reception is cool and the nurse gives the impression of being hurried and uncaring, the patient will react by feeling unhappy and insecure; but the nurse who is warm and welcoming can do a great deal to help a patient to face what, to him, may be an ordeal with greater confidence and peace of mind.

The patient will be asked by the doctor to sign the form of consent for the operation to be performed and will be told on what day and at what time it is proposed that it be carried out. Relatives will want to know details of visiting times and should be given the hospital telephone number, the name of the ward and the most suitable times to enquire on the day of operation. Many hospitals issue a booklet for the general guidance of patients, their relatives and their friends.

The ward sister or nurse admitting the patient should make enquiries about his general health and find out whether he is taking any drugs or is on a special diet, since there may be a general medical condition underlying the local eye condition which has led to his admission. If the patient lives alone or in unsatisfactory home conditions the medical social worker should be contacted so that arrangements can be made for him to spend two weeks at a convalescent home following discharge from hospital. The medical social worker can also help to ensure that when he returns home the services of his Local Authority are mobilized to meet his needs. For example, it may be necessary for home help to be arranged, perhaps the Meals-on-Wheels service and possibly domiciliary nursing care or any other of those services that the Local Authority is empowered to provide.

A thorough general medical examination is made soon after admission, often by the anaesthetist. It may be necessary for the doctor to order certain investigations to be carried out, such as full blood count or chest radiograph. A specimen of urine is obtained for analysis. Occasionally it may be necessary to defer the operation until treatment for an underlying condition has begun. Elderly patients who have been living alone and unsupported may need attention to nutrition, general health and possibly cleanliness before any surgery is undertaken. This will call for tact and sympathetic understanding on the part of the nurse.

Night sedation will probably be prescribed as the anxious patient may find sleep difficult in strange surroundings and amongst strange people.

Instruction in breathing and leg exercises is given to patients by the physiotherapist in order to minimize the risk of such postoperative complications as deep-vein thrombosis, pulmonary embolism and pneumonia.

With the improvement in surgical and anaesthetic techniques and the development of suitable suture materials the use of general anaesthesia has become more common for patients undergoing ophthalmic surgery. In some areas it is still the practice for a local anaesthetic to be used, particularly in those areas where intraocular surgery is carried out in out-patient clinics.

On the day of the operation the patient may or may not be given a light breakfast, depending upon the time of the operation. He is asked to empty his bladder and is then dressed in an operation gown. Any dentures are removed and placed in a labelled container. With women all jewellery should be removed, except a wedding ring, labelled and kept in a safe place; no pins should be left in the hair and all nail varnish should be removed. An identification bracelet is secured on the patient's wrist. The patient who is deaf should be allowed to keep a hearing aid in position until anaesthetized so that he can hear any requests made of him and so that he may feel less cut off from those around him. Premedication drugs are given when prescribed, usually one hour before operation. Preoperative medications commonly used include intramuscular omnopon 10–20 mg with atropine sulphate 0.6 mg. A prophylactic antiemetic may also be given in order to prevent postoperative nausea and vomiting and this may be promethazine hydrochloride 25–50 mg or perphenazine 5 mg. If the operation is to be performed under local anaesthesia, instillation of drops such as procaine 2% should be carried out in the ante-room to the operating theatre.

POSTOPERATIVE CARE

If the patient is unconscious on return to the ward he should be kept under constant observation until normal reflexes return and care must be taken to ensure that a clear airway is maintained. This is achieved by placing the patient in the semi-prone position and supporting the angle of the jaw so that the tongue cannot fall back. When conscious, the patient is asked not to lie on his operated eye and to avoid touching it, as any pressure on the eye may, after intraocular surgery, result in complications such as iris prolapse or aqueous or vitreous loss. Generally little postoperative discomfort is experienced after the majority of eye operations and simple postoperative medications usually prove satisfactory.

The patient admitted for treatment not requiring surgery may find life in the ward very boring. Many such patients are fit and well apart from an eye condition and provision should be made to overcome their boredom. For partially sighted and blind patients, large-type books and tape recorders should be available. Nurses should find time when they can to talk to the patients and fit patients may possibly be allowed to go out for a time during the day with friends or relatives, provided this does not interfere with treatment.

THE CHILD PATIENT

PREOPERATIVE CARE

Most children are admitted to hospital for the surgical treatment of an ophthalmic condition. Sometimes parents and their child may have travelled a long distance to a regional centre equipped to deal with specific conditions. In all cases, it is best that the parents should at least have unrestricted access to the child and where possible arrangements may be made for the mother to remain at the hospital, possibly sleeping in the same room as her small child. It must be borne in mind that when a mother does remain at the hospital, suitable arrangements must be made for the care of any other children remaining at home. The father should be encouraged to visit as often as he is able and his work commitments allow.

Again, it is best if the child can be admitted to hospital 24 hours before operation. When he arrives, a full medical history is obtained by the doctor from the mother, who will remain with the child while a general physical examination is carried out by the doctor. The nurse allocated to care for child and mother will interview them together in order to formulate the nursing care plan which will need to be evaluated fairly frequently, depending on how the child adapts to hospitalization.

The nursing care plan must be explained to the mother as she should be encouraged to help care for her child and will need to be made aware of his special needs.

It may be necessary to use some physical restraint whilst examining the child's eyes, for example wrapping his arms within a blanket, but this should be kept to a minimum and his mother should be close by throughout and able to comfort him when it is over if he is at all distressed. Explanation and reassurance should be given as the examination proceeds.

The child should be weighed as part of the admission procedure in order that the preoperative drugs can be prescribed and the dose calculated according to his weight. A specimen of urine should be obtained for analysis. Before operation he should be allowed to be up and dressed and to play with the other children in the ward. He should also be allowed to keep a favourite toy or object which he has brought with him from home and to take this with him when he goes to the operating theatre.

On the day of operation, if it is to be performed in the morning, it may be necessary to omit breakfast or the 6 a.m. feed, depending upon age, to ensure that no food is given for four hours prior to the administration of the anaesthetic. It will be the nurse's duty, with the mother's cooperation, to make sure that the child has no access to sweets or any other food or drink and that the mother, if present, is warned of the harmful consequences that could follow if he takes anything by mouth.

The premedication will vary according to the wishes of the anaesthetist and must be given at the time stated on the prescription card. The child is then encouraged to settle quietly, where possible with his mother beside him.

POSTOPERATIVE CARE

If the child has not regained consciousness on return to the ward after operation, a clear airway must be maintained, as described for the adult patient, by holding the angle of the jaw forward, and careful observation should be made of his colour and of his pulse and respiration rates.

THE OUT-PATIENT

Ophthalmic out-patient clinics often deal with large numbers of patients, seemingly out of proportion to the number of in-patient beds available. The reason for this is the number of eye conditions which can be treated without the necessity of admission. For some patients this may mean frequent attendances and sometimes daily visits.

Although ophthalmic clinics exist to deal with eye conditions, it is often necessary to subdivide this specialized work further. Patients attend clinics which are arranged for special eye conditions – glaucoma, corneal conditions and so on. The advantage of this arrangement is the more economical use of specialized equipment and personnel.

Many of the people attending clinics are elderly and, particularly if it is a first visit, tend to be confused by the large numbers of people. It is important that the nurse is sure that each patient understands the instructions given to him by the doctor. To help in this, instructions for many simple eye procedures, for example hot spoon bathing or instillation of drops, are printed on cards which can be given to the patient to take home after further explanation by the nurse. The nurse should also make sure either that the patient is able to read the card himself or that there is someone at home who can read it to him and perhaps help with the procedure.

ESTIMATION OF VISUAL ACUITY

When he comes to an ophthalmic clinic or casualty department, the patient's visual acuity will be estimated and recorded. In cases of industrial injury this can be very important if a claim is later made for benefit or compensation. It may be necessary to repeat the test at frequent intervals as a guide to the progress of an eye condition.

The nurse usually undertakes this task and it is necessary for her to become familiar with the various methods of estimating visual acuity, including those used when dealing with young children unable to read or with illiterate patients. Routine testing of distant vision and of colour vision is also carried out by the school nurse employed by a Local Authority as part of the school medical service.

The visual acuity of each eye can be recorded in two ways, for distant and for near vision.

Distant Vision

Distant vision is estimated using a well-lighted Snellen's test type chart (Fig. 1) at a distance of 6 m from the patient. If space is confined the lettering is reversed and reflected in a mirror set at a distance of 3 m;

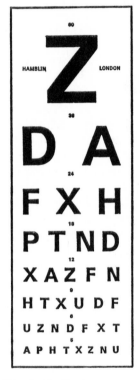

Fig. 1. *Snellen's test types*

the patient then reads the letters reflected in the mirror. The chart consists of a series of letters graduated in size and arranged in horizontal rows. The top letter is of such a size that it can be read at 60 m and the following rows at 36, 24, 18, 9, 6, 5 and 4 m. A person with normal vision can read the sixth line at 6 m and the visual acuity is recorded as 6/6. The upper number indicates the distance the patient is from the chart and the lower the distance at which letters could be read by someone with normal vision. For example, if the reading is 6/24 it is demonstrated that the individual can read at 6 m the letters which a person with normal vision can read at 24 m.

In order to test the visual acuity the subject may stand or sit at a distance of 6 m from the chart; each eye is tested separately (the other eye being covered gently) and the rows are read from above

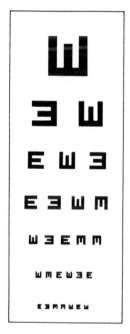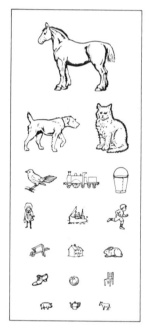

Fig. 2. *'E' test and 'B1474' test types*

down as far as possible, the result being recorded for each eye. If distance glasses are worn, the tests should be carried out first without the glasses and then when they are being worn.

If the top letter cannot be read at 6 m, the distance between the subject and the chart is reduced a metre at a time and the result recorded, for example 3/60 or 2/60. If at 1 m the top letter cannot be read, the person is asked if he can count the number of fingers which the nurse holds up in front of his eyes and against a dark background. If he can do this accurately the vision is recorded as 'counts fingers'

(CF); if not then he may be able to see movement of the hand which is recorded as 'perception of hand movement' (HM). Some patients cannot see hand movements; for them a torch is shone into the eye from different directions. If the patient can tell from which direction the light is coming this is recorded as 'projection of light', but if he can perceive the light only but cannot tell the direction from which it is coming the record of 'perception of light' is made. Before recording the visual acuity of the other eye time must be allowed for the patient to adapt to the light.

Patients who attend an ophthalmic clinic frequently may memorize the test type and a false recording could be made. Most test types are so devised that the chart can be changed. For children unable to read or illiterate patients there are variations to the standard charts. These include numbers, pictures and the 'E' test (Fig. 2); in the latter the child is given a wooden E to hold and point in the same direction as the one on the chart. In the Sheridan/Gardiner test the child is shown letters graduated downwards in size and identifies them by pointing to the same letter on a card that he holds in his hand. In carrying out tests on very young children it is necessary for an assistant (ideally the child's mother) to stand or sit behind him and observe whether he identifies the objects or letters correctly.

Near Vision

Near vision is tested by the patient reading words composed of letters of different sizes, at the normal reading distance of 33 cm. The N series of test types or Jaeger's test type provides the different sizes of printed types. The nurse should ensure that the patient has a good light on the page before trying to read.

PROCEDURES AND TECHNIQUES

Before carrying out any procedure, however simple, an explanation must be given to the patient and he should be made as comfortable as possible so that he is relaxed and as able to cooperate as the circumstances allow. Some procedures are uncomfortable for the patient and others may be rather painful, but if the nurse has been able to gain his confidence various problems can generally be overcome.

SWABBING THE EYES

Though a simple procedure, swabbing the eyes should be carried out carefully, particularly when dealing with an infected eye condition. The requirements include:

Gallipot containing normal saline
Sterile wool swabs
Receiver or bag for soiled swabs

After washing and drying her hands the nurse will stand either behind or immediately in front of the seated patient, whichever is most convenient. Each eye in turn will be swabbed with the eyelids gently closed by the patient first with swabs moistened in the normal saline solution and then, when the eyelids are thoroughly cleansed, with a dry one. The eye should be swabbed from the inner canthus outwards and each swab used once only and then discarded.

INSTILLATION OF EYE DROPS

Instilling drops is a very simple procedure but again one which must be carried out carefully to avoid possible damage to the cornea or contamination of the dropper. Usually one drop of a prescribed substance is instilled into the lower conjunctival sac at one time. If local anaesthetic drops are to be used they are first instilled into the conjunctival sac and then directly onto the cornea.

It is the nurse's duty to check the drops to be used against the doctor's prescription and when drops with antagonistic action are to be instilled into the two eyes of the same patient a second nurse should check the drops and ensure that the correct drop is instilled into each eye.

The patient is either seated comfortably with his head inclined backwards or lying down. The nurse then washes and dries her hands and takes up a position standing either directly behind or in front of the patient. Holding a swab in her left hand and the dropper in her right hand, she will ask the patient to look up, and with the dropper about 2 cm above the eye she will compress the bulb to allow one drop to fall into the conjunctival sac (Fig. 3). The swab is held against the lower lid and the patient is then asked to close his eyes gently; any excess fluid oozing from the eye will be absorbed by the swab and not allowed to trickle down the patient's face. If after the instillation of drops the patient complains of irritation of the skin or of a feeling of heat and tightness the nurse must notify the doctor as this may be an indication of a drug allergy. Should an allergic reaction be confirmed by the doctor this must be recorded in the patient's

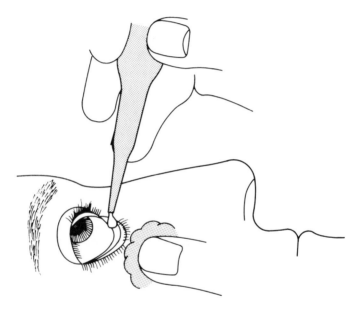

Fig. 3. *Instillation of drops*

notes and the patient himself be made aware of the allergy. If a nurse accidentally instills the wrong drop into a patient's eye it is important that the doctor is informed immediately and the appropriate incident form completed according to local policy.

Eye drops should not be warmed before instillation as the heat may affect the stability of the chemical formula. Commercially packed individual doses of eyedrops should be used in accordance with the manufacturer's instructions. Although the presence of the antiseptic enzyme, lysozyme, in the tears helps to prevent infection it is important that any solution used for treating the eye is sterile.

To prevent the risk of cross-infection, patients either have their own supply of drops in a multiple dose container and disposable droppers are used, or the drops are dispensed in single-dose containers. Multi-dose containers in use within the ward or department must be changed weekly.

INSTILLATION OF OINTMENT

As their absorption rate is less rapid, ointments are used in place of eye drops when a prolonged action is required. They are also used for

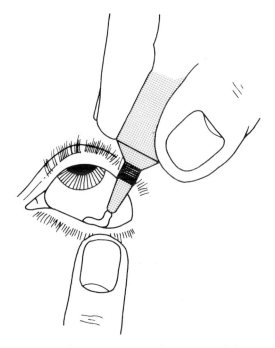

Fig. 4. *Instillation of ointment*

their soothing effect, for example for inflamed lid margins or when the cornea is exposed, as the greasy base forms a protective film over the corneal surface.

Ointment may be instilled from either a multi-dose tube or a single-dose applicator, the latter having the advantage that cross-infection is eliminated. The eye is bathed so that all traces of previously instilled ointment are removed from the eyelids, the patient is instructed to look up, the lower lid is everted (Fig. 4) and a small quantity of ointment is squeezed horizontally into the lower fornix. The patient is then asked to close his eyelids for a few minutes, any excess ointment being removed with a wool swab.

When instilling ointment into the eyes of small children, where any cooperation may be difficult to achieve, the lids must be controlled by the fingers of the nurse and the ointment instilled quickly as the child is attracted to look upwards. Speed is important in dealing with a frightened and possibly struggling child.

With ointment in single-dose applicators, the end of the applicator is cut off and introduced as shown in Fig. 4. If the ointment is packed in a multi-dose tube it is important to avoid contamination of the nozzle.

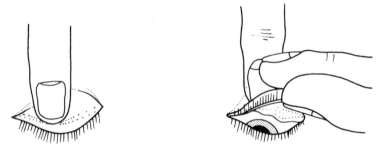

Fig. 5. *Eversion of the upper eyelid*

EVERSION OF THE UPPER LID

The nurse stands behind the seated patient in order to evert the upper lid. The patient is asked to look down whilst the nurse holds the lashes between her forefinger and thumb, the lid is drawn downard and away from the eyeball, a glass rod or the little finger of the other hand is used to depress the upper margin of the tarsal plate and the eyelid is turned over. The lid is kept everted and held gently against the skin, the patient continuing to look down. The retrotarsal space is still hidden and, if necessary, a view of this can be gained by passing a glass rod under the everted lid. This is rather an uncomfortable experience, and to lessen the discomfort a drop of local anaesthetic can be instilled first.

With the experience that comes of practice eversion of the lid may be carried out using only one hand (Fig. 5). This method is useful if it is necessary to evert a lid during irrigation of the eye.

IRRIGATION OF THE EYE

The aim of irrigation is to wash thoroughly the surface of the eyeball and conjunctiva and it may be called for in various situations, as for example when some caustic substance has entered the eye or following silvering of the lids. The apparatus required for carrying out this procedure includes:

Undine—which is kept in a stand when not in use

Jug containing fluid to be used for the irrigation; normal saline is safe and is not irritating to the eye. The temperature of the fluid should be about 37.8°C

Bowl containing warm water in which the jug may stand prior to use

Gallipot containing swabs

Kidney dish or specially designed Fisher's dish to fit against the cheek

Receiver or bag for soiled swabs

Lotion thermometer

Protective cape

The patient may be seated or lying on a couch with his head on a pillow. The protective towel is placed round his neck, covering his shoulders, and he is given the kidney dish (or Fisher's dish) to hold firmly against his cheek on the affected side. The nurse should check that it is in the right position: the head should be tilted a little towards the side. The undine is filled with the lotion at the correct temperature and, after washing and drying her hands, the nurse stands behind the patient, warning him that she is about to begin. She allows a little of the lotion to flow over the cheek to check that the temperature is comfortable to the patient and then, holding the lids apart with the first and second fingers or thumb and first finger, she directs the fluid

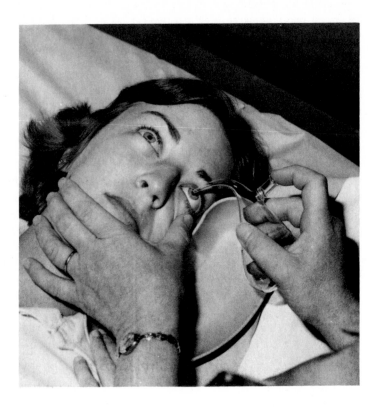

Fig. 6. *Irrigation of the eye using an undine*

in a steady stream over the eyeball (Fig. 6). During the procedure the patient will be encouraged to move his eyes up, down and from side to side. When the undine is empty the eye should be gently dried, as should the cheek before the dish is removed, and the patient made comfortable.

TAKING A CONJUNCTIVAL SWAB

There are two methods used for adults and older children by which the specimen of conjunctival discharge can be obtained.

The easier but possibly less accurate method is the use of a sterile swab on an orange stick supplied by the pathology department. The equipment required includes:

Sterile swab on orange stick
Glass tube
Transport medium

The patient is either seated or lying in bed; the swab is carefully removed from its glass tube, the patient instructed to look up and the lower lid everted. The swab is passed over the exposed conjunctival surface to collect some of the purulent material, after which it is replaced in the tube transport medium, care being taken to avoid any contamination. The swab is labelled and together with the completed request form is sent to the laboratory as soon as possible for incubation on agar in a Petri dish. The label should indicate from which eye the swab was taken and include the patient's name, number, ward and date.

The more satisfactory method employs a platinum loop in place of the sterile swab. The equipment required includes:

Platinum loop
Spirit lamp and matches
Petri dish containing blood agar

The loop is sterilized in the flame of a spirit lamp, allowed to cool and then passed over the exposed conjunctival surface. The nurse then 'plates' the material; the cover of the blood agar plate is removed and the loop drawn across the surface, care being taken not to dig into the agar, and the lid replaced. The agar plate is carefully labelled and placed in an incubator at 37°C for 24 hours. With this method there is no delay in inocculating the plate with the material from the conjunctival sac and a more accurate biological result is obtained. The most common bacteria which may cause conjunctivitis include *Staphylococcus, Haemophilus influenzae, Pneumococcus* and *Neisseria gonorrhoeae*.

The taking of a conjunctival swab from a young child differs in that it requires two people, either two nurses or one nurse and the mother. The equipment required includes:

Platinum loop
Spirit lamp and matches
Petri dish containing blood agar
Blanket

The nurse should wrap the child firmly in the blanket and ensure that both arms are well secured in it. If the mother is remaining with the child she may be able to hold him thus as he will probably be frightened and will feel more secure when his mother is holding him. With the child laid on a cot the nurse (or mother) should hold his head steady with her hands and place her forearms against his arms. The loop is sterilized in the flame of the spirit lamp, allowed to cool and, after the lower lid of one eye has been gently everted, is carefully drawn along the exposed conjunctival surface. The specimen is then plated as before and the Petri dish carefully labelled. It is placed in an incubator at 37°C for 24 hours as with the other specimens. The child is then unwrapped from the blanket and comforted by his mother or the first nurse who should talk quietly to him throughout the taking of the specimen.

HOT SPOON BATHING

Hot spoon bathing is useful in the management of surface infections of the eye lids and is commonly used in the treatment of styes. It helps to relieve pain and causes dilatation of the blood vessels and the increase of the blood supply to the area. Hot spoon bathes should be carried out under the supervision of the nurse, particularly in children and elderly patients when it may be necessary for the nurse to administer the treatment herself. The equipment required includes:

Wooden spoon (not metal as the handle would become too hot to hold) with the neck and tip padded with cotton wool secured in place with a cotton bandage
Bowl or jug containing almost boiling water
Protective towel for the patient's shoulders

The patient sits at a table or, if in bed, uses a bed-table. He dips the spoon into the water, removes excess fluid by pressing the padded back against the side of the container and then brings the spoon as near as is comfortable to the closed lids. He will find that as the water

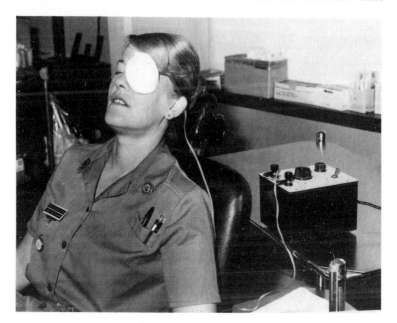

Fig. 7. *An electrically heated eye pad which can be controlled by the patient*

cools he will be able almost to touch the lids; after about ten minutes the apparatus should be removed and the eyelids dried with wool swabs. It is important that the eyelids are kept closed as otherwise the cornea could be damaged. Treatment is repeated two to four times a day.

If the procedure is to be carried out at home, the nurse must make sure that the patient understands what he has to do and if possible a hot bathe should be given in the casualty department by way of demonstration.

A Maddox heater or other small electrically heated pad (Fig. 7) may be used for applying dry heat to the eye. The eye is protected with an eye pad before applying the heated pad. The two pads are then secured in position.

EPILATION OF THE LASHES

Epilation, or removal of a lash or lashes, is carried out for the condition of trichiasis in which the lashes grow inwards and rub the cornea.

The patient should be reassured that although the procedure may be painful momentarily it will be followed by great relief as the cause of the discomfort will have been removed.

The patient is seated comfortably in a chair and a good light is provided. This is necessary because the nurse may fail to see some of the fine lashes that are rubbing the cornea. Special epilation forceps are designed to allow a firm grip on the lash and to prevent it from slipping through the forceps (Fig. 8).

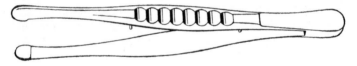

Fig. 8. *Epilation forceps*

The eyelid is slightly everted and the lash is gripped near to its base by the forceps and pulled out sharply. It is necessary to repeat this procedure every four to six weeks as the new lash grows unless electrolysis is used to destroy the hair follicle permanently. If a patient is to undergo treatment by electrolysis the lash must be allowed to become almost fully grown for a satisfactory result.

CUTTING THE LASHES

The lashes are cut in most cases when an eye is to be operated on in order that there is a clear operative area.

A pair of sharp, blunt-ended scissors and a good light are required. Petroleum jelly is applied to the blades with a swab; this causes the cut lashes to adhere to the scissors. The procedure is usually carried out with the patient sitting in a chair, his head supported, or lying in bed with his head on a pillow at the foot end. The upper lid lashes are cut first; the nurse, who stands behind the patient, asks him to look down and, whilst gently holding the upper lid with the index finger of the left hand, cuts the lashes very close to the lid margin. The lashes and petroleum jelly should be removed frequently from the scissors with a swab and more petroleum jelly applied to the blades. The lower lashes are cut in the same way, but with the patient looking up.

Occasionally it may be necessary to irrigate the eye if it is thought that some lashes have fallen into the conjunctival sac. Normal saline is used for the irrigation.

SYRINGING OF THE LACRIMAL PASSAGES

Syringing of the lacrimal sac may be required to determine its patency. Syringing may be carried out by the surgeon, assisted by the nurse, or by a nurse who is experienced in ophthalmology and has been trained in this procedure. As it is difficult to syringe the lacrimal sacs of infants they will require a short general anaesthetic. The equipment required includes:

Nettleship punctum dilator
Lacrimal sac cannula
2 ml syringe
Gallipot
Swabs
Normal saline
Local anaesthetic drops
Fluorescein drops for children
A good light

Before beginning, the patient is given an explanation of what is to happen and is reassured that this is an uncomfortable rather than a painful procedure. However, to help overcome any nervousness and to minimize the discomfort a drop of local anaesthetic is usually instilled near the punctum. It is important for the patient to be warned also that if the sac is patent the fluid may run down the nose and the back of the throat, so there may be a feeling of choking.

The patient is made comfortable either in a slightly recumbent position or lying down with the head well supported; the nurse will check that the syringe (Fig. 9) is filled with the normal saline solution and the cannula is attached.

The patient is then asked to look up and the Nettleship dilator (Fig. 10) is introduced into the punctum; it is passed vertically for about 2 mm and then turned horizontally along the canaliculus. During its passage the dilator is rolled constantly between the thumb and

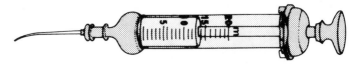

Fig. 9. *Lacrimal syringe*

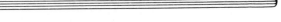

Fig. 10. *The Nettleship dilator*

forefinger. The dilator is then removed and the cannula with attached syringe is introduced in the same direction (Fig. 11). When in position, the plunger of the syringe is slowly depressed; if the sac is patent fluid appears in the nose or runs down the back of the throat at once and the patient will be asked to swallow the salty solution. For small children fluorescein drops may be added and if the sac is patent will stain the saliva.

Attention should be paid to the amount of pressure exerted on the plunger of the syringe. Normally little pressure is required, but if it is found that considerable pressure would be needed an obstruction is present. If fluid, pus or mucus regurgitate the sac is blocked.

RODDING

It may be necessary to carry out this treatment after chemical burns of the conjunctiva to prevent the formation of symblepharon (adhesions) between the lid and the eyeball. The equipment required includes:

Local anaesthetic drops
A smooth, slim glass rod
Sterile petroleum jelly
Swabs

Since this treatment is uncomfortable and painful it is important to instil anaesthetic drops, particularly for the first few days after injury. An explanation of the reason for carrying out the treatment will help to achieve the patient's cooperation and ensure that he returns for as long as is necessary.

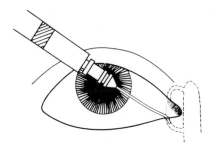

Fig. 11. *Syringing the lacrimal passages*

The nurse should stand behind the seated patient. After instilling the local anaesthetic drops the rod is greased by wiping it with a swab well covered with petroleum jelly. It is then passed under the upper lid and moved from side to side, exerting slight pressure outwards. Any adhesions which are forming are broken down and a film of grease left between the two surfaces. Atropine or an antibiotic ointment may be prescribed and sometimes used in place of petroleum jelly.

SUBCONJUNCTIVAL INJECTION

As the conjunctiva is connected very loosely to the underlying tissues the introduction of drugs between these layers will allow better absorption. Examples of drugs given by subconjunctival injection are mydriatics, antibiotics and steroid preparations. The mydriatic drug Mydricaine is of great value in iritis when other methods of dilating the pupil have failed.

If possible two nurses should carry out this procedure, one to instil the anaesthetic drops and hold the light and the other, an experienced nurse, to give the injection.

When the procedure is explained to the patient he should be told to expect pressure as the conjunctiva balloons up when the drug is injected. No pain should be felt except when antibiotics are injected; for this a small amount of procaine 2% may be injected first.

After the eye has been anaesthetized the patient is asked to look up and the needle (size 20) is inserted into the conjunctiva below the limbus, avoiding any obvious blood vessels. Alternatively the fluid may be injected into the excess folds of conjunctiva in the fornices. The fluid is injected steadily, causing the conjunctiva to balloon. The point of the needle should always be visible and no more than 1 ml of fluid should be injected at any one time. The needle is removed and the patient asked to close his eyes gently, as squeezing will cause the fluid to leak out. A pad and bandage are applied and the patient given whatever analgesic has been prescribed.

The site of the injection is always near to the affected area, but the lower segment is preferred as surgery may be planned in the near future and if the incision is to be made in the upper segment it could be complicated if this was the site of a recent conjunctival injection.

3

Eye Drops and Medications

The nurse working in an ophthalmic unit should be familiar with the action of the commonly used eye drops and ointments. She must also be able to instruct patients clearly and concisely how to use these at home.

Drugs for use in the eye are classified according to their action:

1. Mydriatics and cycloplegics.
2. Miotics.
3. Antimicrobials.
4. Anti-inflammatory drugs.
5. Local anaesthetics.
6. Diagnostic stains.
7. Miscellaneous.

MYDRIATICS AND CYCLOPLEGICS

Mydriatic drugs dilate the pupil by affecting the dilatory and con-tracting muscles of the iris; cycloplegics paralyse the ciliary muscles and prevent the process of accommodation of the lens. Drugs which fall into this class have differing durations of action, lasting from half an hour to several days. Thus the selection of the appropriate treatment for a particular patient will depend upon the type of action required:

1. Short-term dilatation of the pupil for examination of the eye.
2. Longer-term treatment for uveitis, keratitis, iritis or iridocyclitis.
3. On occasion, after operative treatment or accidental trauma.

Atropine, as 1% eye drops or ointment, is the most commonly used mydriatic. Dilatation of the pupil occurs half an hour after instillation, but accommodation is not paralysed until about two hours have elapsed. The mydriatic effect of atropine may last for more than a week and cycloplegia for two to four days, therefore for diagnostic purposes the shorter acting drugs, homatropine or cyclopentolate, are preferred. Apart from its shorter duration of action (onset of mydriasis from 15 to 30 minutes, lasting from six to 24 hours), homatropine has the added advantage that, unlike atropine, its effects may be readily reversed by the action of physostigmine. The mydriatic effect of homatropine is enhanced by cocaine and the two drugs are sometimes used together.

Cyclopentolate (Mydrilate), from which full recovery of accommodation occurs within 24 hours, has become one of the most useful drugs for refraction. Toxic effects are uncommon, although central nervous system disturbance has been reported.

On occasion it is necessary to give a mydriatic by subconjunctival injection; for this a combination of atropine sulphate and cocaine, known as Mydricaine, is used.

Drugs may be absorbed through the eye and the use of atropine should be avoided in babies who may also be receiving the drug by injection preoperatively: the total amount received from both routes of administration could constitute an overdose.

In some patients atropine may cause conjunctival irritation; atropine-like substances may also cause tachycardia, disorientation and ataxia. In these people an alternative mydriatic should be used; this may be one of the following: hyoscine, lachesine, cyclopentolate or phenylephrine. Lachesine eye drops 1% are a useful alternative for patients who are intolerant of atropine or hyoscine; phenylephrine 10% drops, although they cause irritation and must be used in conjunction with a local anaesthetic, are of value when mydriasis without cycloplegia is required.

Mydriatics should not be used in patients with glaucoma as they may increase the intraocular pressure. For elderly patients, in whom the drainage angle may be partially blocked because of sclerotic changes, the prolonged use of mydriatics, particularly atropine, may precipitate an attack of glaucoma, the dilated pupil further reducing the already incompetent drainage of aqueous.

Patients with dilated pupils will experience some degree of photophobia and if the eye is uncovered the patient should be advised to wear dark glasses. If both pupils have been dilated for examination of the fundus in the out-patient department, the action of the mydriatic should be reversed by a miotic or the patient detained until the effect of the eye drops has worn off. This is particularly important for a patient who is driving a car.

MIOTICS

Miotics are drugs which have the opposite action to mydriatics: they constrict the pupil and contract the ciliary muscle. Thus they are used to counteract the action of mydriatic and cycloplegic drugs used for examination of the eye. Reversal of the action of mydriatics is especially desirable in those over 40 years of age because of the positive danger of precipitating an acute attack of glaucoma.

Miotics increase the aqueous outflow through the filtration angle and trabecular meshwork and are used in the treatment of glaucoma.

As with the mydriatics, the miotic group of drugs comprises compounds with varying onset and duration of action and the choice of miotic will depend upon the effect desired.

In the management of glaucoma the selection, strength and mode of use of miotics is dependent upon the intraocular pressure and its response to previous therapy. Frequent measurements are made so that the patient's treatment may be adjusted to give the optimal reduction in pressure.

The most commonly used miotics, both in the treatment of glaucoma and in the reversal of mydriasis, are pilocarpine and physostigmine (eserine). The strength of the eye drops prescribed may vary from 0.25 to 1.05% in the case of physostigmine (or 1% if only eye drops are used) and from 1 to 4% in the case of pilocarpine.

Pilocarpine has the shorter duration of action of the two and is relatively free from side effects. When used in concentrations greater than 0.25% physostigmine may be an irritant. The two drugs are sometimes used in combination as they have a synergistic action.

Two other miotics which are used less frequently are ecothiopate (phospholine iodide) and dyflos (DFP). Both these drugs have a very powerful, long-lasting effect but their use is limited by their side effects; they have a tendency to irritate the eye and DFP may cause visual blurring, severe pain and frontal headache. Both should be used with extreme caution where there is a history or suspicion of retinal separation. DFP is the only miotic capable of reversing the effect of atropine.

ANTIMICROBIALS

Antimicrobial drugs for use in the eye are normally applied topically, as eye drops or eye ointments, but occasionally subconjunctival injections are used.

The choice of drug will depend upon the infecting organism. Sometimes, as in the case of an infection with herpes simplex, a specific antimicrobial drug, idoxuridine, must be used, as this virus will not respond to other drugs. More frequently broad-spectrum antibacterials, which are active against a number of organisms, are prescribed; chloramphenicol and neomycin are examples of antibiotics used in this way.

ANTI-INFLAMMATORY DRUGS

Corticosteroids have anti-inflammatory activity no matter what the cause of the reaction. They may be used systemically in eye disease, but if possible local treatment with drops or ointment is employed. Hydrocortisone, prednisolone or betamethasone are the steroids most frequently used in the eye.

Steroids should not be used when bacterial infection is present unless the patient is having adequate antimicrobial treatment as well. Their use during viral infection of the eye is contraindicated as they encourage viral replication and render the infection worse.

The indiscriminate use of steroids should be guarded against as, apart from the complications already mentioned, use in the presence of severe corneal ulceration may cause thinning and perforation, while prolonged use may raise the intraocular pressure in some patients who are predisposed to glaucoma.

Antihistamine eye drops, such as antazoline, are sometimes prescribed for allergic inflammatory eye conditions but they are not as efficient as corticosteroids.

LOCAL ANAESTHETICS

Many procedures require the prior instillation into the eye of a local anaesthetic; for instance cocaine eye drops, 2–4%, are employed before the removal of foreign bodies. After the use of cocaine the anterior aspect of the eye remains insensitive for at least half an hour. Cocaine causes a slight mydriasis and drying of the corneal epithelium and it is advisable that the eye be covered until the effect has worn off. Other local anaesthetics in use as eye drops are amethocaine and lignocaine which, although less effective than cocaine, do not have its disadvantages and can be used prior to tonometry. Procaine 2% is used when infiltration of the eye with a local anaesthetic is necessary.

DIAGNOSTIC STAINS

Corneal damage, either from an ulcer or following trauma, is more readily assessed if a stain or dye is instilled into the eye before examination. Fluorescein, the stain usually employed, outlines the disrupted epithelium with a pale yellowish-green colour and Bengal rose dyes the tissues rose pink in the damaged area.

MISCELLANEOUS

Methylcellulose and, more recently, hypomellose eye drops are used as artificial tears. Less viscous drops are used for lubricating contact lenses and a more viscous preparation is instilled before gonioscopy to prevent the formation of air bubbles.

PRECAUTIONS

It must be understood that the introduction of contaminated eye drops or ointment into a diseased eye may result in an infection which could lead to the loss of the eye. Thus it is important that sterility is maintained, especially when the eye is damaged when any organism inadvertently introduced can penetrate the tissues. When using diagnostic stains the nurse is by definition putting drops into an eye suspected of being damaged. For this reason fluorescein drops should be used once only from single-pack sterile containers. When multi-dose eye drop bottles are used for continued treatment, for example with atropine or hydrocortisone and neomycin, each patient should have an individual container and this should be renewed as frequently as indicated by the hospital pharmacy.

Occasionally patients may have an adverse reaction to a drug used locally in the eye. This may be irritant, as in the case of atropine eye drops, or allergic, as sometimes happens with the use of neomycin. Any worsening of inflammation in the eye or spread of inflammation to the surrounding skin should warn the nurse that the patient may have a drug reaction and the treatment should be stopped, the doctor being informed at once. It is generally possible to find a substitute therapy which the patient will tolerate.

Though these questions of sterility and possible adverse reactions are also discussed in Chapter 2, describing nursing procedures, their importance cannot be over-emphasized.

4

The Lens

The lens lies in front of the vitreous body and behind the iris. It is a soft, transparent, biconvex body enclosed in a thin homogeneous capsule. The central points of the anterior and posterior surfaces are known as the anterior and posterior poles and a line taken through them is known as the axis. The anterior surface of the lens is in close contact with the pupillary margin of the iris and the central part of the lens is opposite the pupillary opening. Towards the periphery, the lens is separated from the iris by the aqueous in the posterior chamber. The close contact of the iris with the lens can be demonstrated in a patient who has had a heavy blow to the eye, for example with a football: on slit-lamp examination iris pigment which forms a ring corresponding to the pupil may be seen on the anterior lens capsule. A slit-lamp is shown in Fig. 13.

The posterior surface of the lens is more convex than the anterior surface and occupies the hyaloid fossa of the vitreous body.

The lens is composed of a series of concentric lamellae of fibres, the edges of which are connected by a cement-like substance, enclosed within a thin capsule. This capsule is a transparent membrane which closely surrounds the lens and is thicker on the anterior surface. The capsule is formed early in fetal life, probably as a secretion from the epithelial cells which form the lens vesicle in the embryonic fetus. The function of the capsule is to mould the lens and protect its substance from the vitreous and the aqueous; it also plays an important part in accommodation. An explanation of the mechanism of accommodation is given on p. 36.

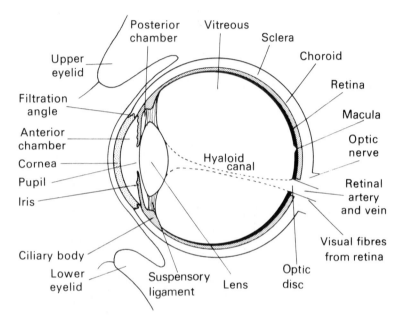

Fig. 12. *Section of the eye*

The lens is retained in position in front by the pressure of the aqueous humour (the physiology of which is very similar to cerebrospinal fluid) and behind by the vitreous humour which is a clear, transparent gel-like substance filling the space between the posterior surface of the lens and the inner surface of the retina, and by the zonule or suspensory ligament. This is a delicate membrane which covers the inner surface of the ciliary body and processes and the lens surfaces.

The physical characteristics of the lens vary at different periods of life. In the fetus it is nearly spherical and rather soft. In the adult the anterior surface is less convex than the posterior surface and its substance is firmer. From about 40 to 45 years of age the lens increases in size, is flattened, assumes a yellowish tinge and becomes tougher, and these changes constitute the condition of presbyopia, which is described on p. 39.

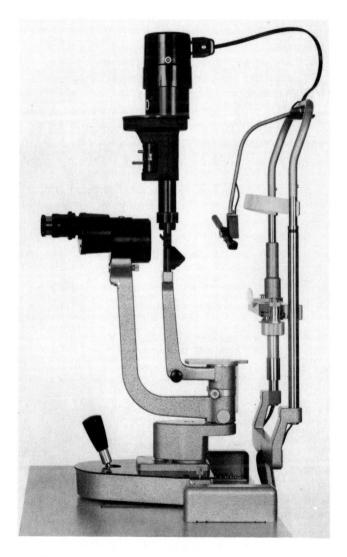

Fig. 13. *The Haag–Streit slit-lamp microscope with R900 attachment*

REFRACTION OF LIGHT

The lens plays an important part in the refraction of light.

Refraction is the deflection of light when it enters obliquely a medium of different density, for instance as from air to water. This can be demonstrated easily by placing a ruler in a jug of water. The ruler looks bent at the surface of the water. As the rays of light pass from the air through the transparent structures of the eye known as the refractive media, the rays are bent. The refractive media include the cornea, the lens and the vitreous. The lens is important in this process as it bends the light rays in order that they can be focussed on the retina. From the retina the light is converted into light impulses which are transmitted via the optic nerve to the centre of sight in the occipital lobe of the brain.

If the lens stayed at a fixed focal length the image would be blurred when the object was brought close to the eye. To enable close objects to be seen clearly some change must take place in the convexity of the lens to alter the focal length. This process is known as accommodation. Accommodation is possible because of the zonule or suspensory ligament which surrounds the lens and which is controlled by the ciliary muscle. When the ciliary muscle contracts, the suspensory ligament relaxes, increasing the lens curvature. This is accompanied by some convergence of the eyes and constriction of the pupils to enable light rays to pass through the central portion of the lens. In the normal eye it is possible to see objects as closely as 25 cm away. Closer work requires the use of a special lens such as that used by a watchmaker. Refraction of rays of light of near and far objects is shown in Fig. 14.

ERRORS OF REFRACTION

Emmetropia

Normal sight, emmetropia, occurs in a nearly spherical eye where the vertical and transverse diameters are only 1 mm shorter than the anterior –posterior diameter (Fig. 15A).

Errors of refraction are due to abnormalities in the form of the eyeball.

Myopia

In myopia (short sight) the anterior—posterior diameter is abnormally long and since parallel rays of light are brought to focus in front of the retina, diffusion circles will form only a blurred image upon the retina (Fig. 15D). The myopic eye often appears to be larger than the normal eye.

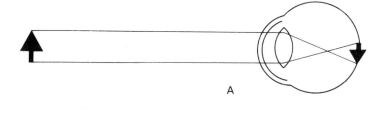

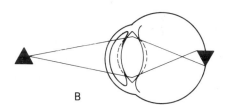

Fig. 14. *Refraction of rays of light. A, From a distant object, more than 6 m away, rays are parallel. B, From a near object, less than 6 m away, rays radiate from every point*

Myopia is rarely congenital although there may be a strong hereditary tendency, particularly in some people such as the Chinese and the Jews. It commences at an early age, is often progressive and in a small percentage of cases may lead ultimately to retinal degeneration or even detachment. However, in the majority of cases myopia worsens only through the growing years and may then improve slightly in later life. Retinal detachment is discussed in Chapter 5.

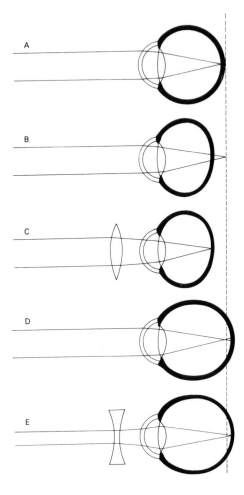

Fig. 15. *Errors of refraction. A, A normal emmetropic eye:
parallel rays are brought to focus on the retina. B, A hypermetropic
eye: the eyeball is too short and the rays are brought to focus behind
the retina. C, Hypermetropia is corrected by a convex converging lens.
D, A myopic eye: the eyeball is too long and the rays are brought to
focus in front of the retina. E, Myopia is corrected by a concave
diverging lens*

Hypermetropia

In hypermetropia (long sight) the anterior—posterior diameter of the eyeball is short and the image is brought to focus behind the retina (Fig. 15B). The refracting power of the lens is not sufficient to converge the rays acutely enough to form a clear image on the retina.

There are also hereditary tendencies in this condition. Correction is achieved by means of convex lenses which converge the rays before entering the eye, so aiding the effect of the crystalline lens.

Astigmatism

Refractive error brought about by irregular curvature of the cornea is called astigmatism; the rays of light enter in different planes and are brought to focus at varying distances from the retina. This is usually a congenital condition and is present to some degree in all eyes; only when it is well marked can it be considered abnormal. Astigmatism may be acquired as a result of inflammation, injury or operation on the cornea.

The condition is treated by giving the lens an added convexity or concavity in the appropriate meridian since astigmatism may be associated with myopia or hypermetropia. Vision improves after the lenses have been worn for some time and so spectacles or contact lenses should be worn constantly.

Presbyopia

A defect of accommodation, presbyopia develops from middle age. The lens loses its elasticity with advancing years and there is an inability to focus on near objects, whilst distant vision is not affected. Convex lenses are required for reading ordinary print.

Whilst most refractive errors are corrected by spectacle lenses, contact lenses are becoming more popular (see pp. 56–60), particularly in the correction of myopia. However, some patients may not easily tolerate wearing contact lenses and dislike the idea of using them so that the choice, where it is applicable, should be left to the individual.

CATARACT

Cataract was the name applied to the condition of lens opacity centuries ago when the loss of vision was thought to be caused by a 'curtain' which fell down over the inside of the eye, rather like a waterfall.

Cataract is largely a disease of the elderly but may also be congenitally determined, presenting either at birth or later during the developmental process. Other factors concerned in the production of cataract include disease, particularly diabetes mellitus, some vitamin deficiencies, notably vitamins B1, B2 and C, and trauma. In tropical countries it is thought that ultra-violet light may be partly responsible for the formation of cataract and it is also thought that undue exposure to heat or cold may be possible factors to be taken into account.

SENILE CATARACT

The type most commonly found is senile cataract and it is a degenerative process. The changes associated with presbyopia occur, the lens becomes less transparent and tougher, but in addition it becomes yellow in colour and opaque. The opacity prevents refraction of light.

Although referred to as a senile cataract, the changes may begin to develop early in middle age; by the age of 70 years the majority of individuals have some lens changes, which may, however, cause only slight difficulty with vision.

The onset of the condition is gradual, with a slight impairment of vision which becomes progressively worse. The length of time which may elapse before a person seeks medical advice depends to some extent upon his occupation; for example, a draughtsman or an electrician may notice a deterioration in his sight sooner than a builder's labourer.

Diagnosis of cataract can be established quickly as it is possible to see the changes in the lens by the use of an ophthalmoscope. However, it is very important to assess the general physical health of the individual and also to determine whether there are any other reasons for loss of vision.

It is usual for the patient to be seen in the first instance by his general practitioner who will have a knowledge of his previous medical history and who, after explaining to the patient what in his opinion is the most likely cause for his failing vision, will refer him to an ophthalmologist.

On the first visit to the ophthalmic clinic the patient's visual acuity is assessed and this is repeated on subsequent visits. The patient is received by the nurse in the clinic and, if any explanations or instructions given by the doctor are not clearly understood by the patient, it will be her duty to make sure that he does understand what is going on and what may be expected of him.

Details of the patient's general health are obtained and carefully recorded as these may affect the timing of his future admission to hospital, when this is necessary. Where there is a history of chronic bronchitis the patient is usually admitted for lens extraction during the summer months if possible in order to lessen the danger of coughing postoperatively. A diabetic patient may need to be assessed by the physician before admission for surgery. The incidence and progress of lens changes in the elderly appear to be greater when diabetes mellitus is present. Hypertension, deafness and the possibility of a brain tumour should also be watched for and it is often routine for urine analysis and estimation of blood pressure to be carried out and for any abnormalities to be referred to the physician in order that treatment may be given before admission for surgery. During all these investigations, and if referral to the physician is necessary, the nurse can support and reassure the patient and do much to allay any fears he may have.

At this first visit careful examination of the eye is carried out, to include the condition of the eyelids, the cornea, the depth of the anterior chamber and the pupil.

The pupil is usually dilated by the instillation of a mydriatic, for example atropine sulphate 1%. Mydriatics, as well as dilating the pupil, are also usually cycloplegics, that is, by paralysis of the ciliary muscle they prevent the lens from being able to accommodate for near vision. When the nurse is instilling the drops she should stand behind the seated patient, gently pull down his lower lid and instil the drops into the outer side of the lower fornix. The purpose of dilating the pupil is to make it possible to assess the state of the lens, as in some instances the changes may be at the periphery. An attempt is made to examine the fundus in a darkened room with the aid of an ophthalmoscope.

If the lens is completely opaque the state of the retina cannot be seen and to determine whether or not the retina is functioning a simple test can be carried out. An explanation is given to the patient who is seated in a darkened room with the less affected eye covered. A light is then shone into the other eye from various angles and the patient is asked to indicate the direction from which the light comes. If he is correct it can be assumed that the retina is healthy and the following symbol:

is used to denote accurate perception of light in all quadrants.

After the ophthalmologist has assessed the patient's condition, he discusses the findings with him. If the patient's normal activities are not hindered too much then he is reassured and asked to return at regular intervals for observation of the cataract. Patients who have opacities in the centre of the lens may gain benefit from the use of such mydriatic drops as homatropine which enable them to see through the clearer periphery of the lens. Here the nurse should satisfy herself that the patient is able to instil the drops himself or has someone who can do this for him. For some people, a change of spectacle lenses may give temporary improvement of vision. As soon as the patient is unable to continue his everyday activities, then admission to hospital for lens extraction is advised. Development of the cataract is gradual and will vary with the individual so that it is not possible to predict with any accuracy when an operation will be required.

Preoperative Care

The patient admitted to the hospital for lens extraction should be made to feel welcome to the ward and as much at home as possible. He will be introduced to his fellow patients who will usually be able to give him a good deal of information regarding the ward routine, how to use the trolley telephone, how to obtain any necessary items and so on. (A more detailed description of this procedure is given in Chapter 2.) If vision is very poor, the patient will need even more careful orientation to his new surroundings by the nursing staff.

The principles of the nursing care of patients undergoing lens extraction may be applied with slight modification to other types of intraocular surgery. The patient is prepared as for any other operation and usually also for a general anaesthetic. The nurse should spend some time with the patient, telling him what is going to happen and why and doing her best to overcome any fears he may have in regard to the successful outcome of the operation.

In addition to the usual preparations certain special preparations are necessary. Following an examination of the eyes, certain routine treatments will be commenced. These vary according to the wishes of the surgeon, but are likely to include the following procedures. A conjunctival swab may be taken (see p. 18) of both eyes to exclude the presence of pathogenic organisms in the conjunctival sac. Cutting the lashes of the eye (see p. 22) to be operated on is undertaken in order that there is a clear operative area. This procedure may produce some anxiety in the patient owing to the presence of the scissors so close to the eye; in very nervous patients and in children it may be necessary to cut the lashes in the anaesthetic room when anxiety has been inhibited by the premedication drugs given or even in the theatre itself after the patient has been anaesthetized. It is also important to reassure the patient that the lashes will have grown again in about three weeks.

Syringing the lacrimal ducts (see p. 23) may be carried out as a blocked duct may be the source of pathogenic organisms for which treatment will be required preoperatively. In such a case antibiotic drops are instilled into both eyes four times daily.

Local preparation on the day of operation includes instillation of drops to ensure that the pupil of the eye for operation is fully dilated to allow access to the lens. A combination of swift-acting, short-duration mydriatics is employed, the particular drug used being that preferred by the individual surgeon. The reason for this is that although dilatation of the pupil is essential during the operation, postoperatively it is undesirable as it may cause the vitreous to prolapse into the anterior chamber or may precipitate a prolapse of the iris through the wound.

Vasoconstrictor eye drops may be instilled to reduce the risk of operative haemorrhage, together with a mydriatic. If local anaesthetic drops are also used the eye must be padded as the cornea will be insensitive to foreign bodies and it will also become dry. The nurse from the ward will accompany the patient to the anaesthetic room, taking with her his notes, and will remain with him until he is anaesthetized. The patient at this time will be drowsy and probably experiencing some degree of euphoria as a result of premedication, but the nurse should talk quietly to him, explaining what is going on in order to 'take his mind off' his strange surroundings. This is particularly important with children who are of an age to appreciate their situation and with the elderly who may be feeling confused and, if the operation is to take place under a local anaesthetic, frightened.

The Operation

During the operation the operating theatre nurses will be responsible for seeing that everything is prepared correctly; individual surgeons may vary in the instruments they use and the way they carry out their work. The nurse who is 'scrubbed' will hand the instruments to the surgeon in the correct order and see that he has everything as he needs it. A second nurse who is not scrubbed (but who, like everyone else in the operating theatre will be wearing appropriate clothing to minimize any risk of infection) will act as 'runner' to fetch any further articles that may be required and generally look after the scrubbed nurse and the surgeon and his assistant. Where the operation is being carried out under local anaesthesia, it is essential there should be quiet as a sudden noise might cause the patient to move. If possible a nurse, preferably the ward nurse, should sit by the patient, holding his hand, and talk to him quietly and as far as she can constantly reassure him. Some patients undergoing surgery under local anaesthesia may appreciate a background of soothing music.

Extraction of senile cataract may be achieved by removing the contents of the lens without the capsule, by removing the contents with the capsule or by phakoemulsification.

Extracapsular lens extraction   A limbal or corneal incision is made and the anterior lens capsule is ruptured. The solid lens is then expressed from the eye through the wound and any remaining soft lens matter is washed out with saline. If left it will cause a uveitis; that is inflammation of the pigmented layer of the eye comprising the iris, ciliary body and choroid. The remaining posterior lens capsule may require needling or capsulotomy some weeks or months later since the posterior capsule may become wrinkled or thickened by the adherence of residual lens matter. This involves making a hole in the capsule to provide clear vision. This is a safe operation as it avoids disturbance of the vitreous and the possibility of loss of vitreous through the wound.

Intracapsular lens extraction In this operation both the lens and the capsule are removed together. A variety of techniques have been developed for this procedure which include the use of non-cutting

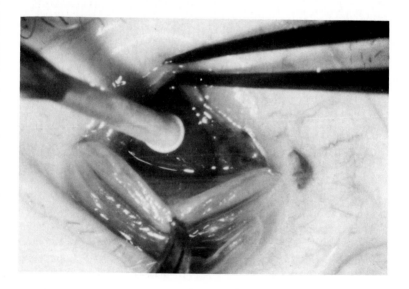

Fig. 16. *Lens extraction using a cryoprobe*

forceps, removal of the lens by suction using an erisophake and the use of a freezing probe or cryo (Fig. 17). The use of an enzyme α-chymotrypsin behind the iris a few minutes before the removal of the lens, by partially digesting the zonule of the lens, facilitates its dislocation from its zonular attachment to the ciliary body, without rupturing the capsule. The advantage of intracapsular lens extraction is that there is no need for a second operation and it is usually the method of choice. However, there is a greater risk of vitreous loss and in patients who are myopic and are more susceptible to vitreous loss, an extra-capsular lens extraction may be preferable.

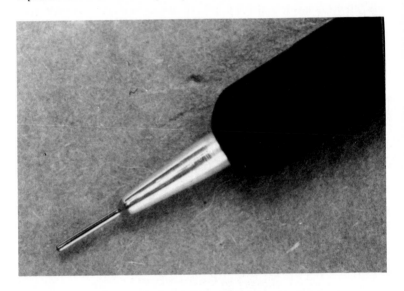

Fig. 17. *The cryoprobe used for lens extraction*

Since in senile cataract the lens is hard and sometimes swollen, it may be necessary to make an incision as large as half of the circumference of the cornea. This may be achieved in various ways and more recently a corneal section is made, but this requires the use of an operating microscope. The main advantage of this method is that there is no operative haemorrhage. In removal of the lens one or two peripheral iridectomies, that is the provision of one or two small holes in the peripheral part of the iris, may be performed and in some cases a large iridectomy may be necessary to prevent a postoperative rise in intraocular pressure which may occur when the iris is resting on the vitreous.

Careful suturing avoids distortion of the cornea and astigmatism and also prevents the formation of a shallow anterior chamber caused by a leaking section. As atraumatic sutures are now readily available, which enable the surgeon to suture securely, the postoperative in-patient period has been shortened.

Phakoemulsification This achieves lens removal through a small 2 mm incision, reducing postoperative complications and hospitalization time. A 1 mm vibrating tube is held against the lens and small particles of the lens are detached and immediately aspirated. This method is not as yet in general use.

With improved anaesthetic techniques, the majority of operations are now carried out under a general anaesthetic. A local anaesthetic is sometimes used when the patient's physical condition does not warrant the use of general anaesthesia.

At the conclusion of the operation a dressing is applied to the eye, usually consisting of tulle gras, and an eye pad secured with Sellotape. A cartella shield may be used to afford added protection to the eye.

Postoperative Care

In the majority of instances the patient is conscious on return to the ward. Care must be taken to place him gently in his prepared bed. Beds where the head can be detached make this procedure easier, as do 'rollers'. If there are no special instructions, the patient is made comfortable with two pillows. If a patient is unconscious on return to the ward he should be placed on his side, with the operated eye uppermost to lessen the risk of damage to it, and should be kept under constant supervision as is the case in any patient unconscious after anaesthesia.

The aim during postoperative nursing care is to allow full healing of the wound: every effort must be made to avoid anything which may delay this such as restlessness, vomiting or coughing. The importance of rest and quiet during this critical period will have been explained to the patient and the nurse will do everything she can to enlist his co-operation and to reassure him. If both eyes are bandaged the patient will have no vision at all and he must be able to feel that the nurse is near or easily summoned and that she will make sure that he has everything he needs. His bell should be within reach and his locker placed by his bed on the side of the unoperated eye when the operation has been unilateral. His fellow patients will also most likely be very helpful at this time. Any postoperative restlessness or nausea should be relieved by the administration of the sedative or antiemetic ordered.

During the first postoperative day, in order to avoid vigorous movement, the bed is only tidied, particular care being taken to ensure that the bottom sheet is smooth and comfortable. The patient is washed by the nurse, his pressure areas are treated and he is given a urinal or bedpan as necessary, the nurse being especially careful when moving him for these purposes and enlisting the help of a second nurse if required. The patient's hair is not brushed or combed until after the first dressing of the eye; cleaning of the teeth and, in the case of male patients, shaving are also deferred until then. Oral toilet will be carried out gently by the nurse if the patient complains that his mouth is dry. The patient is encouraged to rest and sleep for most of this day.

If the patient has reasonable vision in the unoperated eye he is allowed to feed himself, otherwise the nurse must feed him. Aperients are best avoided at this stage and as constipation may occur because of the patient's dislike of using a bedpan it may be advisable to take him to the toilet in a sanichair if the need arises.

Visitors may be allowed for a short period provided they understand the necessity for the patient to be quiet and to avoid all unnecessary movement.

The first postoperative dressing is usually carried out 18—24 hours after operation in the presence of the surgeon. The trolley is prepared, the blinds in the ward are drawn if it is a very bright day. The patient is told what is going to happen and is asked to put his arms inside the bedclothes; this is to avoid the possibility of his touching his eye or the dressing.

Any bandage is removed and the adhesive material holding the pad in position is cut. If the pad is not stuck to the lids it is removed; if it is adherent a swab should be moistened at the tip with normal saline and, with a pair of forceps, the pad is peeled off from above downwards, the swab steadying the lid. Meanwhile the person undertaking the dressing will have washed and dried her hands, opened the dressing pack and put a sterile towel on the pillow and shoulders of the patient. Lint or wool swabs are used, moistened in normal saline. Some surgeons insert a suture in the upper lid which is secured to the cheek by Sellotape; this suture will be cut near to the skin of the lid, the stitch drawn out and then cut near to the strapping on the cheek. The eye is then swabbed very gently without exerting any pressure, from the medial to the lateral canthus. Each swab is used once only, inspected for discharge or debris and then discarded. It should be remembered that the patient's other eye, even when it has not been operated on, will also require swabbing and this may be done first to accustom the patient to the sensation.

After the lids are thoroughly cleansed the patient is asked to open both eyes; a swab is held against the cheek to catch the overflow of tears which occurs when the operated eye is opened for the first time. A careful examination of the anterior segment of the eye is then made.

The cornea should be clear and bright although some striate keratitis (inflammation of the cornea, causing cloudiness) may be present as a result of handling of the cornea. The anterior chamber should be reformed, though any presence of blood (hyphaema) should be noted. Hyphaema is caused by bleeding from the iris or the edge of the incision into the anterior chamber and in other circumstances may occur spontaneously or as the result of a knock on the eye. The pupil should be round and central; distortion may be the result of an iris prolapse through the wound. The patient is asked to look down and, if the upper lid is gently drawn up, the wound can be seen. When the patient opens his eyes for the first time he will notice how bright things appear. A patient who has previously been short sighted may be able to see clearly as the lens extraction will correct previous visual defect. Many patients may be disappointed and despondent because they do not see so well at first; this may be due to many factors including striate keratitis and lens matter left in the eye. These patients will need encouragement and reassurance that, when the eye has settled, improvement will take place.

Sometimes antibiotic drops are instilled at the first dressing and occasionally mydriatic drops to dilate the pupil and rest the iris. The eye is gently dried and a fresh pad applied. The opportunity can be taken by the nurse to comb the patient's hair; this should be done very gently as tugging at any snags will be detrimental to the healing of the wound.

Provided the first dressing is satisfactory, the patient is allowed out of bed for a short time. As bending the head forwards causes pressure

on the suture line, the patient is asked to avoid bending and stooping.

On the second postoperative day the patient is given a full bed-bath
and is then allowed to sit in a chair. A normal diet may be taken.
Patients may walk to the toilet, with help if necessary, and, as many
patients undergoing this operation will be elderly, they may need
support and assistance in walking and any other independent movement. On the third day the patient may have a bath in the bathroom
under the supervision of a nurse, but if he is rather infirm a bath in
bed may be preferable. On this day an aperient can be administered
if it is needed. The patient, although more ambulant, must still take
care to avoid stooping.

The eye is dressed each day and on the third to fifth day the pad is
removed; dark glasses are worn during the day and the eye is padded
at night. If the patient has previously had a lens extraction in the other
eye and has spectacles designed for aphakic correction—that is for
correction of an eye from which the lens has been removed—then
for that eye he may wear these spectacles with the addition of dark-
tinted clips to reduce the light glare, which he may find troublesome.

Patients who have no vision in their unoperated eyes are given
temporary cataract spectacles to which they find difficulty in adjusting
at first, but which they soon manage very well. These temporary spectacles allow the patients wearing them to be more independent whilst
they await their own individually prescribed spectacles. In the majority
of cases the patient is ready for discharge from hospital on the fifth
to seventh postoperative day. Preceding discharge a thorough examination of the eye is carried out using a slit-lamp microscope which
gives a good view of the section and the anterior chamber.

Patients are given out-patient appointments for 7–10 days later,
but if they are worried about their eyes they should return earlier.
They may also be given drops to instil, with further careful explanation
and instruction, and the nurse may suggest that if possible another
person should instil the drops. Patients must be advised to avoid any
heavy lifting and stooping for another two weeks. Women are often
anxious to have their hair shampooed; this may be done a few days
after discharge from hospital and a backwash at the hairdressing salon
is preferable to bending forwards over a basin. Before elderly patients
leave hospital the ward sister should satisfy herself that home conditions

are satisfactory, if necessary enlisting the help of the medical social worker in order that the services of the local authority and voluntary organizations may be called upon where necessary.

Postoperative complications both of the eye itself and more generally are now less frequent as a result of advances in surgery and early ambulation. Frequent attendances at the out-patient department are necessary in the first six weeks after discharge to ensure that the eye settles with no complications such as anterior uveitis, aphakic glaucoma or aphakic detachment of the retina. After six weeks a refraction is carried out. The prescribed glasses are thick convex lenses which are a substitute for the natural lens; this makes the spectacles rather heavy, with a tendency to slip down the nose. Two pairs of glasses are necessary, one for near and one for distant vision. Some patients may ask for bifocal lenses. Contact lenses can be fitted after cataract operation on one eye only when the use of a contact lens will make the images sufficiently near the same size to enable both eyes to be used together again. Contact lenses are discussed on pp. 56–60.

CONGENITAL AND DEVELOPMENTAL CATARACT

A congenital cataract is present at birth and a developmental cataract occurs in the early years of life as the result of a congenitally determined defect. These forms of cataract may be caused by hereditary, toxic, nutritional or inflammatory processes. Perhaps the best known example is the cataract which may occur in the infant when the mother has contracted rubella in the first eight weeks of pregnancy. This condition is usually bilateral and results from the toxic effects which take place during the time of the development of the eyes in the embryo. Maternal rubella in the first trimester of pregnancy may affect other organs, for example the infant may also be found to have a congenital heart lesion. A child with congenital cataracts will need to be admitted to hospital for treatment and two or more admissions may be needed at close intervals. Binocular congenital cataracts should be removed by needling, in which the capsule of the lens is torn with a special needle, within a few months of birth if they are severe enough to render the infant blind and so prevent the development of macular fixation; otherwise, or if only one eye is affected, a needling is generally carried out at about the age of six years.

Preoperative Care

In addition to the general preparation of the baby or child for operation and anaesthesia there must be special preparation of the eye.
After admission a swab may be taken of the lower conjunctival sac
for culture and a sensitivity test of any pathogenic organisms. To
obtain a conjunctival swab from a young child is a simple procedure
technically and is described on p. 20. If pathogenic organisms, such
as the *Staphylococcus aureus*, are grown the surgeon may consider
postponing the operation and will institute a course of antibiotic eye
drops. In any event, after the conjunctival swab has been taken the
child may be given a course of antibiotic drops six hourly as a prophylactic measure. To instil drops into the eye of a child under two years
of age it is necessary to restrain him in the manner described for taking
a conjunctival swab (see p. 20). However, older children, after the procedure has been explained, will usually be cooperative without any
restraint being used.

It may be repeated here that, where possible, and providing the local
conditions of the hospital allow, it is desirable to allow the mother to
remain with her child during his stay in hospital. To do so is likely to
lead to far less emotional trauma which may persist after his return
home and in addition many mothers can be of great assistance to the
nursing staff by carrying out their normal care of their own child. If it
is not possible for the mother to be with her child then unrestricted
visiting should be allowed and positively encouraged.

On the day of the operation mydriatic drops are instilled. These
are prescribed because it is essential to ensure that the pupil is fully
dilated in order to give the surgeon clear access to the lens.

The Operation

The method for removing congenital cataract (also traumatic cataract
in the young) is discission or needling. The operation involves making
a large hole in the interior lens capsule with a capsulotomy needle;
this allows the soft lens matter to escape into the anterior chamber
where it is either aspirated through a small corneal wound, using a
syringe and needle, or left for natural absorption of the lens matter

to take place. This operation may need to be repeated several times.

Postoperative Care

The child will be received into his prepared bed and cared for under close supervision until he has regained consciousness, if he is not already conscious on return to the ward. When a young child goes to the operating theatre he will often take with him a familiar object or toy which is very important to him and he should find this beside him when he recovers from the anaesthetic.

It is now more usual to leave the unoperated eye uncovered and for the operated eye to be covered with an eye pad secured with adhesive tape.

The child is usually kept in bed for the first 24 hours as too much activity may precipitate bleeding from the iris and a hyphaema. The first postoperative dressing is performed by the doctor who, after gently swabbing the eye with normal saline, will wish to examine the eye for signs of any free lens matter or blood in the anterior chamber and to observe the size of the gap made in the lens capsule. Mydriatic and antibiotic eye drops are usually instilled. After the first dressing it is often more satisfactory to leave the eye uncovered as an eye pad often causes young children irritation and they rub the eye under the pad.

A toddler is allowed up on the second day and may join in play activities in the ward. Eye drops are instilled daily and the eye observed for any complications; these may be synechiae (adhesion of the iris to the cornea in front or to the lens, where it is present, behind), glaucoma caused by malabsorption of the lens matter or a persistent hyphaema. The child is discharged from hospital three to five days after operation and the mother is given an appointment to bring him to the out-patient department a week later.

When all the soft lens matter has been removed, the child will need to be supplied with spectacles to compensate for the lack of natural lenses. These are usually well accepted even by very small children, who wear spectacles with extended sides through which ribbon is threaded and the glasses tied in place.

TRAUMATIC CATARACT

Any break in the lens capsule as a result of injury, for example a perforating injury of the eye caused by a sharp instrument, may result in cataractous changes. If there is a large opening made in the lens capsule, aqueous will enter and this will cause absorption of the lens. Liberated lens matter may cause a uveitis. Operative treatment is necessary.

Uniocular cataract which may follow trauma often results in the patient finding he has difficulty with spectacles after operation. The spectacle lens for aphakic correction will give up to 20% magnification whilst the other eye is normal. This may cause diplopia (double vision) and for these patients contact lenses may be prescribed.

For some patients an artificial lens (Fig. 18) made of an inert plastic substance is inserted into the eye. These intraocular artificial lenses are inserted into the anterior chamber either between the iris and the vitreous or suspended in front of the lens when the eye has settled after lens extraction.

This may cause some irritation to the eye with postoperative iritis which usually settles. If the eye will not tolerate the lens and does not settle the lens can be removed. Research is being undertaken to produce an intraocular lens which will be readily accepted by the eye. The lens has the same refractive power as a human lens but cannot accommodate for near objects and so reading glasses are necessary. Postoperative care for these patients follows the pattern of care after lens extraction (see p. 47).

DIABETIC CATARACT

Diabetic cataract is less often seen today as there has been an increasing emphasis on the need for early diagnosis and treatment of diabetes mellitus. Some general practitioners carry out routine screening tests on the patients on their lists who are aged 60–65 or over and some local authority clinics also screen the elderly for this and other conditions. However, diabetic cataract sometimes occurs in adolescent patients with this disease.

Senile cataract in diabetic patients is similar to that in non-diabetic subjects, but the incidence is higher in the diabetic patient and the condition tends to develop more rapidly.

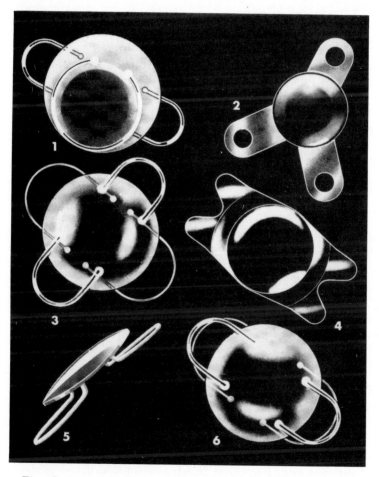

Fig. 18. *Intraocular lenses in current use. 1, The Worst two-loop implant. 2, The Rayner Pearce tripod posterior chamber lens. 3, Iris lens clip. 4, The Rayner Choyce anterior chamber implant. 5, The iridocapsular lens, after Binkhorst. 6, The iris lens clip, after Binkhorst*

COMPLICATED CATARACT

Complicated cataract may occur following a long-standing ocular disease such as uveitis, glaucoma or retinal detachment and may also be seen in patients with intraocular tumours; such cataracts seldom warrant removal.

CONTACT LENSES

Contact lenses are so named because they are in direct contact with the outer surface of the eye. Types in use at present include the following:

1. *Corneoscleral or haptic lenses* fit over the cornea and sclera, although only the corneal section of the lens provides refractive correction. These lenses, although they are bulky, cannot fall out and are easier for poorly sighted patients to handle. This type of lens is used mainly for the diseased eye and needs specialist fitting. They are also used by people who indulge in vigorous sporting activities. They are likely to exert some pressure on the veins which drain the aqueous and so produce a rise in intraocular pressure in patients with a narrow drainage angle (see Chapter 7).

2. *Microcorneal lenses* are the size of the patient's cornea; they are less bulky, being made as thin as possible, more comfortable to wear and do not affect the intraocular pressure. However, they do fall out more easily and may cause ulceration of the limbus.

3. *Soft lenses* are a recent development. They are made of softer materials resembling gelatine, but are as thin as the other types of contact lens. They are made from several plastic or rubber-like materials which have a water-absorbing property and for this reason are suitable only for patients with sufficient tears. In addition, coloured eye drops and those containing drugs should not be instilled into an eye containing a soft lens. In certain conditions the water absorption property of the lens can be used to advantage; a soft lens may be inserted to avoid repeated instillation of drugs, e.g. of pilocarpine in the treatment of glaucoma. They may also be used to protect a desensitized cornea, hold mucous membrane grafts in position and for the correction of errors of refraction.

A soft lens is usually more easily tolerated than other types of contact lens and children readily adapt to them following surgical treatment for congenital cataract. The development of these lenses

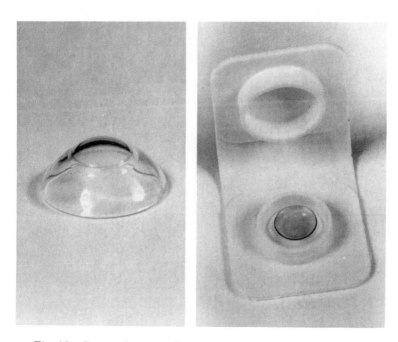

Fig. 19. *Contact lenses.* **Left,** *Scleral (haptic) lens.* **Right,** *A hard corneal lens in a mailing case*

is still in process; at present they wear out after several months, the time depending upon the degree of handling and trauma to the lens. Storage and handling of the lenses are important; they should not be allowed to dry out and handling should be reduced to a minimum. The hands must be thoroughly washed and all traces of soap removed before handling a soft lens.

When removing the lens, the patient is asked to tilt his head backwards and look up. The lens is gently slid downwards using the index finger on to the bulbar conjunctiva, it is then lifted off the conjunctiva with the thumb and index finger.

The patient is taught how to fit his contact lenses and he will soon develop techniques for insertion and removal of the lens. Various solutions may be used with which to insert the contact lens, but normal

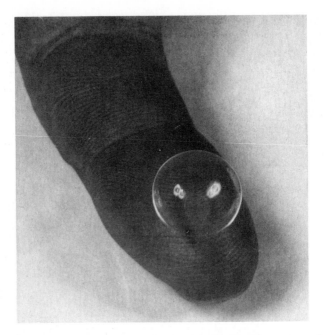

Fig. 20. *A soft contact lens balanced on a finger prior to insertion. The white marks are reflections of the camera flash*

saline is probably as satisfactory as any. Some patients are excessively sensitive to the presence of a lens in the eye and may need to be very persistent and determined in order to learn to tolerate it. Contact lenses can be worn without discomfort from three to six hours, although many patients can retain them in position for the whole day. Hard contact lenses should not be worn during sleep, but some soft lenses may be worn continuously except for occasional cleaning. The nurse must be able to remove a contact lens if the patient has a painful cornea ulcer when he may be unable to do this for himself. One common method is to use a small rubber suction pad, supplied with hard lenses, for both insertion and removal. To remove the lens if the eye is painful the patient should be seated and a few drops of a local anaesthetic

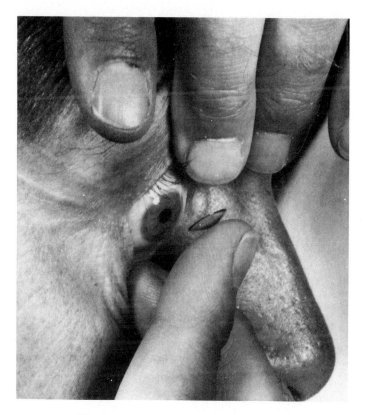

Fig. 21. *Insertion of a hard corneal lens*

instilled. The patient is then asked to look downwards. The suction end of the rubber cap is moistened and the air squeezed out. The upper eyelid is then retracted gently and the cup applied to the upper surface of the lens. The pressure of the suction holder is released and the lens will then be lifted downwards and out over the lower lid. Any corneal condition must heal completely before the lenses are worn again.

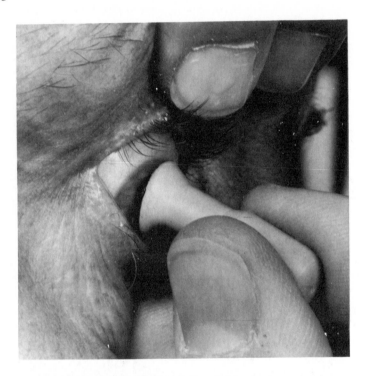

Fig. 22. *Removal of a scleral (haptic) lens using a sucker*

Care of contact lenses is important, as they are delicate and require careful handling. They are supplied in a special box with full instructions as to their care. Since the microcorneal lenses are necessarily very small, great care must be taken not to drop them when they are being inserted or removed as it may be very difficult to find them again.

5

The Retina

The retina forms the innermost layer of the eye and is referred to as the light-perceiving layer. It is a soft, delicate, thin membrane which in the living eye is transparent. The thickness of the retina gradually diminishes from 0.4 mm near the entrance of the optic nerve to 0.1 mm at the ora serrata, its anterior extremity. It is purplish-red in colour because of the visual purple, or rhodopsin, in the rods which with the cones make up the outer layer of the optical part of the retina. The retina is placed between the hyaloid membrane of the vitreous internally and the choroid externally. The inner surface of the retina has a 'yellow spot' or macula lutea about 1−2 mm in diameter which is the area of the most distinct vision. About 1 mm to the nasal side and slightly below is a whitish disc which appears slightly raised and corresponds to the entrance of the optic nerve; this is the optic disc. This area consists only of nerve fibres which are insensitive to light and which is known as the 'blind spot'.

In the detailed complex structure of the retina, shown in Fig. 23, the light-sensitive elements consist of this specialized layer of rod- and cone-shaped cells. The rods are used when the light intensity is low and give a grey picture. They are densely crowded at the front of the retina. They convert the light stimulus into a volley of electrical impulses which travel along the sensory nerves to the visual area of the brain. For this function rhodopsin is required. The pigment is slowly broken down as it absorbs light of low intensity and the breakdown releases the energy which triggers off the nerve impulses. The function of the pigment cells found next to the choroid is the renewal of rhodopsin. Rhodopsin is a substance composed of protein and the pigment

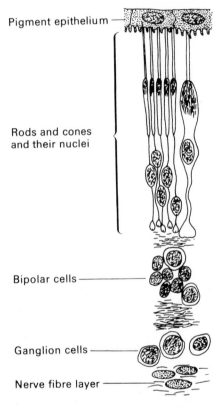

Pigment epithelium

Rods and cones
and their nuclei

Bipolar cells

Ganglion cells

Nerve fibre layer

Fig. 23. *Cross-section of the retina*

carotene; this compound when bleached by light rays splits, and the pigment is converted into vitamin A. In the dark rhodopsin is resynthesized from vitamin A and protein.

The other receptors in the retina, the cone-shaped cells, are used in daylight vision and are responsible for the appreciation of colour. The cones are confined to the central regions of the retina. Sensitivity to different colours is not uniformly distributed over the retina, the area sensitive to blue is the largest and that sensitive to red next in order of size.

DARK–LIGHT ADAPTATION

When one enters a dark room from a light one it is momentarily impossible to see; after a time objects can be perceived dimly and then become more distinct. Dark–light adaptation is brought about by increased sensitivity of the rods as a result of regeneration of rhodopsin with dilatation of the pupils which allows more of the available light to enter the eye. Conversely, the dazzling effect of bright light after being in the dark occurs because the eyes have adapted to dim light. Light adaptation is caused by the bleaching effect of light on the rhodopsin with reduced sensitivity of the rods and constriction of the pupil which restricts the amount of light entering the eye.

THE VISUAL PATHWAYS

Nerve impulses from the retina are transmitted along the optic nerve to the brain. The fibres of the optic nerve, forming the innermost layer of the retina, converge at the optic disc and then pierce the outer layers of the retina. The optic nerve is about 4 cm long and passes backwards and medially through the back of the orbital cavity; it then runs through the optic foramen into the cranial cavity and joins the optic chiasma. At this point the nerve fibres from the medial side of the retina cross to the opposite side and join the fibres from the lateral side of the retina which remain on the same side. These fibres form the optic tract and pass through a 'relay station', the lateral geniculate body, to the visual cortex of the occipital lobe of the brain. The visual pathways are shown in Fig. 24.

The left side of the visual field is seen by the right half of the eyes and conversely the right side of the visual field by the left half of the eyes; in the normal eye the visual areas of the brain fuse the two separate images transmitted to them from both eyes to form one single mental impression of the object viewed.

Damage to the optic nerve would result in blindness in the affected eye. If nerve fibres at the optic chiasma are subjected to pressure such as that from a pituitary tumour this may cause blindness of both

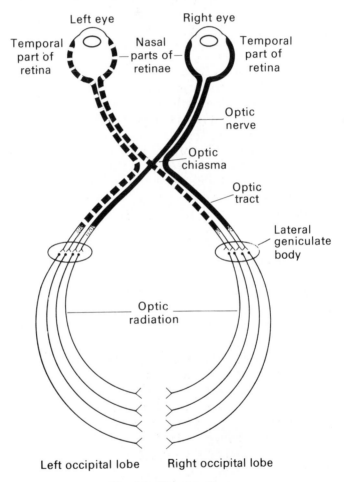

Fig. 24. *Visual pathways*

temporal fields of vision or total blindness. Pressure or damage in the optic tract will also affect vision in both eyes, but the nasal fields will be affected.

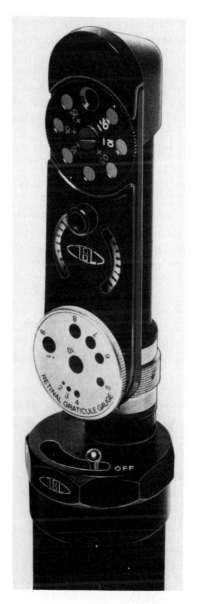

Fig. 25. *A direct ophthalmoscope*

Wherever possible the nurse should be given the opportunity to use an ophthalmoscope in order to view the retina and to identify the main structures. An ophthalmoscope is an instrument with which to illuminate the retina using a battery and a small bulb (Fig. 25). For normal vision the ophthalmoscope has a small hole through which to look; lenses are provided to fit into the aperture to correct focussing defects when either the observer or the subject normally wears spectacles.

When the retina is viewed through an ophthalmoscope (Fig. 25) the macula can be seen as a small oval area devoid of blood vessels; blood vessels can be seen leaving the optic disc. A normal fundus is shown in Plate I/1.

Electrodiagnostic instruments have been introduced to aid detection of conditions of the choroid and retina when dense opacities of the refractive media prevent viewing with an ophthalmoscope. An electroradiogram measures the electric potential of the retina; an electro-oculogram records the changes of ocular potential due to metabolic activity.

Pathological conditions of the retina present either with a sudden, painless loss of vision or with a long-standing visual loss that may be so gradual in its onset that it is not noticed by the patient. Separation of the retina is the most common of these conditions.

A proportion of patients with retinal changes are referred to the ophthalmologist from medical clinics, for example hypertensive patients with retinal degeneration and those suffering from diabetes mellitus in whom, especially the elderly who may have been treated for many years, retinal changes are almost always bilateral.

RETINAL DISORDERS

CENTRAL RETINAL VEIN THROMBOSIS

Central retinal vein thrombosis (Plate I/3) is associated with arteriosclerotic changes. The patient has sudden but incomplete loss of vision and multiple haemorrhages can be seen over the retina. Anticoagulant drugs are of little value. Although the condition does appear to improve in time, new blood vessels sometimes form which block the drainage angle and this may lead to glaucoma (raised intraocular pressure).

CENTRAL RETINAL ARTERIAL THROMBOSIS

Sudden and total loss of vision caused by central retinal arterial thrombosis (Plate I/2) unfortunately is usually irreversible by the time the patient is seen as the retina will die in three to four minutes when deprived of its blood supply. This condition may occur in the elderly person but is also seen in young adults with bacterial endocarditis when emboli break off and reach the retinal artery. If it is possible to undertake treatment immediately the clot may be dislodged by vigorous massage of the eye or by a paracentesis (tapping) of the anterior chamber which will result in a sudden reduction in the intraocular pressure, dilatation of the blood vessels and the dislodging of the clot.

The central artery of the retina, together with the vein, pierce the optic nerve about 11 mm from the globe and pass between the bundles of nerve fibres to the inner surface of the retina near the middle of the optic disc. There is a central depression in the optic disc, the optic cup; gradual enlargement of the optic cup may be seen in patients with raised intraocular pressure.

COLOUR BLINDNESS

An inherited defect in the cones causes colour blindness. It is most usually found in males and is frequently first detected during testing for colour blindness in routine school medical examinations. As colour blindness most commonly affects the ability to distinguish between red and green it may be a bar to certain occupations where normal discrimination of colours is essential.

RETINITIS PIGMENTOSA (PRIMARY PIGMENTARY
DEGENERATION OF THE RETINA)

Retinitis pigmentosa is a slow degenerative disease of the retina usually occurring in both eyes and being hereditary. The most characteristic symptoms are night blindness and complaints of failing vision in poor lighting conditions. Degeneration is first seen to occur in the rod cells; retinal pigmentation develops and gradually encroaches upon the retina, with eventual constriction of the retinal blood vessels and development of lens opacities. The onset is often during the early 'teens, with gross handicap occurring in middle or advanced age. No

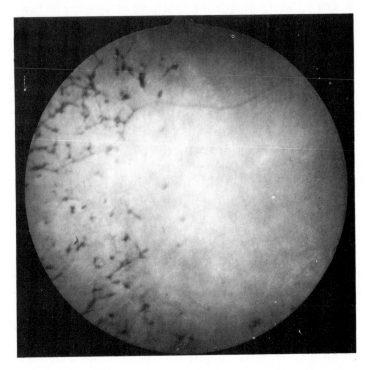

Fig. 26. *Retinitis pigmentosa, showing the peripheral 'bone corpuscles'*

treatment is available but the patient may be prescribed some aids to help with mobility until blindness is total.

SOLAR RETINOPATHY

Solar retinopathy occurs when the unprotected eye is exposed to the bright sun and can result from looking at an eclipse of the sun. Exposure to the infra-red rays causes a burn on the retina. At times when an eclipse of the sun is expected people are advised to view it through smoked glasses.

Eye injury may result in contusion of the retina (commotio retinae). This usually follows a blunt injury and is often associated with a traumatic hyphaema. The retina on the area opposite the injury becomes oedematous; retinal changes and retinal holes may occur. Patients with this condition are admitted to the ward for about one week. During a period of rest in bed careful observation of the retina is made for any changes which may take place and the hyphaema is treated either by rest alone and sometimes also by the application of heat by means of an electric warmer (see Fig. 7).

RETINAL SEPARATION

The condition which is often called 'detachment' may more accurately be described as 'separation' of the retina, since where there is a breach in the retinal tissues fluid accumulates between the layer of rods and cones and the pigment epithelium of the retina. This can happen because the outer layer of the retina (the pigment epithelium) and the inner layer (the optical parts) lie in apposition without any form of union except round the optic disc and at its wavy border, the ora serrata. Thus primary retinal separation occurs when any cause, such a breach, allows fluid from the vitreous to seep into the subretinal space. Primary separation of the retina may follow injury to the eye or myopic changes or it may be idiopathic. In myopic patients retinal separation occurs usually between 30 and 40 years and is more common in men than in women. Those people where myopic changes more commonly occur, for example Jews, have a higher incidence of retinal separation, although it is interesting to note that the Chinese, who are also often myopic, rarely develop retinal separation.

Separation of the retina may also occur as a secondary manifestation, when no tear is present, in many conditions, of which toxaemia of pregnancy, retinal retinopathy and a mass in the choroid are examples.

In primary separation of the retina there is no pain and thus the patient may not seek medical help at the outset. When seen by a doctor some patients complain of flashes of light, the result of stimulation of the loose retina as the eye is moved; others describe the loss

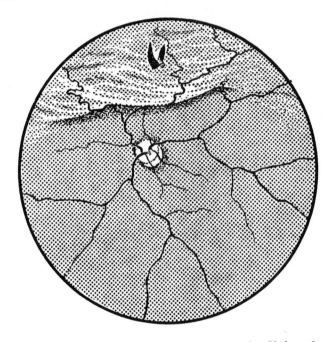

Fig. 27. *Retinal detachment in association with a U-shaped tear*

of vision as a shadow starting somewhere at the side of the field of vision and increasing in size. It should be noted that separation is a gradual condition starting often at the periphery where the retina is thinnest and extending gradually until the affected eye is totally blind. This process may take only days or may extend over weeks and months.

On examination with the ophthalmoscope the retina will present a dull grey colour and may be in folds. Holes and breaks may be visible; these may take the form of U-shaped tears (Fig. 27) or round holes or the retina may be torn away at the ora serrata. Once a diagnosis of retinal separation has been made the patient should be admitted to the hospital ward. This may come as a considerable shock to the patient, who is usually in good general health, and there will be anxiety concerning the sudden loss of sight and the prospect of two or three weeks in hospital. The nurse must be aware that the patient may have these feelings, which can present themselves as frank anxiety, disbelief or even open hostility, and she must be prepared to deal with the patient in a sympathetic and understanding manner so as to give him the maximum reassurance. The patient will also be apprehensive because the successful outcome of surgery cannot be guaranteed and in some cases later admissions to hospital will be required for further surgery. It is important that considerable time is taken to explain carefully the reasons why admission is essential, the treatment which is planned, the possible outcome of that treatment and the general regimen that will be followed.

The doctor will have talked to the patient in the first place and told him all this, but the nurse will be responsible for ensuring that the patient really understands what he has been told, since in his confusion and anxiety he may well not have appreciated much that has been said. Patients may suffer bouts of depression, especially if they fear that vision will be reduced permanently. They may also, naturally, wonder whether the same fate may eventually overtake the other eye, leaving them totally blind. Thus the nurse must be ready to give constant support to such patients and be willing to give as much reassurance as she can at this stage.

Prognosis

While about 75% of all separated retinas can be replaced, the factor essential to a more positive prognosis is *time*. The chances of a successful replacement in a case left untreated after a year would be worsened significantly. Unsuccessful results after treatment would require further surgery in about three to four weeks and in such cases the ultimate prognosis is even less good.

Preoperative Care

Patients admitted to hospital for surgery following retinal separation are usually encouraged to rest in bed for a few days prior to operation.

The position in bed will depend upon the area of separation, but those with a superior retinal separation should be positioned with the separation at its lowest point; for example, if the upper and outer area of the right eye is separated the patient should lie on his right side with the foot of the bed raised. This allows the retina to settle, prevents further separation and encourages the absorption of fluid which has seeped beneath the retina. The position is not very comfortable, but if it is explained to the patient why it is necessary it will be easier for him to accept. It may be necessary in these cases to nurse him at complete bed rest, so that he is fed and bathed by the nurse, or it may be permissible for him to get up for toilet purposes and to sit up for eating his meals, returning to the original position between these times.

On the other hand, where the lower half of the retina is separated the patient will be nursed propped up with pillows in a sitting position.

It is now rare for patient to have both eyes padded and occluded glasses are more commonly worn to discourage eye movements. The instillation of mydriatic drops to both eyes paralyses the muscles of accommodation and provides a widely dilated pupil for the viewing of the retina through the ophthalmoscope.

During the period of waiting for surgical treatment and immobility a mild sedative may be necessary to help to relieve anxiety and to control restlessness. Night sedation is also often needed.

The length of time between admission to hospital and operative intervention varies considerably. During this time careful drawings will be made of the retina to show the position of holes and degeneration and the extent of the separation, and these will be referred to throughout the operation. The usual preoperative investigations are carried out and should include urine analysis and a full medical examination. Preoperative medication will be ordered.

In addition to an understanding and sympathetic attitude by doctor and nurses every care should be taken to meet the patient's social and psychological needs. Visitors will bring news of family and friends and provide contact with the world outside hospital; they may read books or the newspaper to the patient. The radio may be a source of enjoyment and distraction from his troubles and conversation with ambulant patients may help to prevent boredom.

The Operation

The aims of surgery will be: (*a*) to release the subretinal fluid, (*b*) to seal the holes or tears and (*c*) to create an internal ridge to which the retina will adhere (shortening the eyeball).

The subretinal fluid is removed by making a small hole through the sclera, the tough, white, outer layer of the eye.

Much progress has been made recently in the ways in which the sealing of the holes can be achieved. In one method surface diathermy is applied to the sclera overlying the area of the tear. The diathermy causes a reaction and union of the choroid and retina in the area of the diathermy so that the hole is obliterated. During this procedure the surgeon frequently has to verify the correct position of the diathermy applicator.

A less damaging method of sealing the holes is by the application of intense cold using the cryotherapy retinal probe to a temperature of -80°C. The advantage of this method is that postoperative adhesions are less likely to form.

A more direct method is the use of a light coagulator (photocoagulation) with a very strong beam of light directed through the pupil which welds the retina on to the choroid. The only disadvantage of this method is that for it to be successful the retina must be in close apposition to the choroid with no subretinal fluid present.

The laser beam provides a reaction similar to the photocoagulator but with a greater accuracy. Recent developments have seen the laser beam used in the out-patient department, with only local anaesthetic to the surface of the eye required. This form of treatment is especially useful as a palliative measure in patients with small weakened areas of the retina which, without treatment, may result in retinal separation.

Shortening the eyeball may be achieved by various methods, the most common of which is to encircle the eye around the equator (the midportion of the eye) with a silicon rod or strap. This is particularly useful in patients with myopia or an aphakic detachment when there is shrinking of the vitreous. Small local plombs of silicone may be buried under the sclera to cause a local indentation.

Postoperative Care

The patient is received into his prepared bed in the way usual for all patients following general anaesthesia and is kept under close observation if and for as long as he is unconscious. His position in bed is again dependent upon the site of the retinal detachment and the position adopted should be maintained for four to ten days. During this time the nursing care is similar to that for a patient after a lens extraction (see Chapter 4). However, since the trend is now towards early ambulation, the nurse must be able to adjust the nursing care to accord with the wishes of the surgeon. It is now unusual for the patient to remain with both eyes padded and after the first dressing dark glasses are usually allowed.

Some patients, particularly those who have had an encircling procedure, complain of some ocular discomfort similar to neuralgia which responds well to a simple analgesic such as paracetamol.

During the period following operation and before discharge every effort should be made to prevent the patient feeling bored and depressed. The radio again will be enjoyed by many, talking books may be used, visitors will help and usually will be awaited eagerly and the nurse should spare time whenever she can to talk to the patient and, if he wishes it, discuss his progress with him in the light of what she has been told by the ward sister and has read in the ward reports. Generally speaking, patients are discharged from hospital two weeks after surgery with an appointment to return to the retinal clinic in 10–14 days. Checks by the ophthalmologist will then be advised at increasing intervals until ultimately examination every year or two will be sufficient. The patient should be advised to avoid stooping and heavy lifting and should perform only light tasks for some weeks after operation. If he is normally engaged in heavy manual work it may be necessary to look for some lighter alternative with the assistance of the medical social worker and, where necessary, the Disablement Resettlement Officer of the Department of Employment. With elderly patients, perhaps living alone, arrangements should again be made in conjunction with the local authority for help to be provided in daily living. It may well be that home help and Meals-on-Wheels will be required.

RETINOBLASTOMA

Retinoblastoma is a malignant neoplasm of the retina, often of congenital origin. It may be present at birth or first become apparent in early childhood. It may be hereditary. The tumour can be fairly well advanced when first noticed by the parents as a white mass behind the pupil giving the appearance of the 'cat's eye reflex'. Sometimes it is detected earlier if the infant or child is examined by an ophthalmologist for a squint which arises as a result of loss of vision in the affected eye. If the condition occurs in one eye where there is a family history it is likely that the other eye may become involved.

In order to confirm the diagnosis the pupil is dilated by the instillation of mydriatic drops and the eye examined using an ophthalmoscope. In the early stages treatment can be carried out successfully by the application of radioactive cobalt plaques over the site of the growth and of the optic nerve. For very small malignancies light coagulation therapy may be used in conjunction with cobalt therapy. Where the condition is in an advanced stage, however, the only treatment is enucleation (removal) of the affected eye, together with as much of the optic nerve as possible.

Preoperative Care

Many problems confront the nurse who is dealing with a child admitted to hospital for enucleation. Often the parents may have travelled a considerable distance to a regional centre equipped to deal with this condition; they will be extremely anxious and, if a family history of retinoblastoma exists, may have feelings of guilt. Such parents will need a great deal of help to deal with their emotions and will also need practical advice and help in deciding whether the mother is to remain with the child in hospital (where this is practicable), the care of any siblings left at home, possibly help with fares for frequent visiting when the mother must leave the child. It may be possible for the local authority at home, working in conjunction with the hospital medical social worker, to arrange for temporary admission of any siblings under five to a day nursery run by the social services department who, alternatively may be able to supply such help as a home maker who will look after the children and the home for as long as is necessary.

The child may settle quite well, but the parents will need constant support and reassurance; although the doctor will have explained the nature of the disease and its implications it is usually to the nurse that they will confide their fears and of whom they will ask their questions. The nurse must always be ready to deal with the parents with tact and sympathy and must be able to tolerate any episodes of hostility caused by possible feelings of guilt and inability to accept the catastrophe that has befallen their child.

Postoperative Care

If cobalt plaques are applied the postoperative phase can be rather trying for the child. There is usually severe chemosis (oedema) of the conjunctiva and some local discomfort. The child usually feels unwell and unhappy.

Regular gentle cleansing of the eye is essential. Although games which can be played in bed should be provided these should be simple and of short duration as the child will tire easily. After an enucleation has been carried out the child may appear much brighter. This is especially so if the tumour has caused a rise in intraocular pressure and thus discomfort. Children usually accept the fitting of a glass shell or temporary artificial eye very well, but much patience and tact may be needed when instructing the parents in the care of the shell as they find the procedure unpleasant and difficult to accept.

When the socket is healed and the child discharged the parents must understand the need for the frequent reviewing of the condition. Follow-up at the clinic will be at monthly intervals at first and then the time between visits is gradually increased. It is essential that regular examination is made to rule out the presence of any secondary deposits of the tumour or any involvement of the other eye. The parents should also be advised that any other children should also be examined in order to exclude the presence of a tumour in their eyes and it may be advisable for genetic counselling to be given since the children of a further generation are at risk and must be examined from early infancy. Where necessary the question of special schooling for blind or partially sighted children may be discussed.

If a child misses an appointment at the clinic for any reason the parents must be contacted and another appointment made. This can be done direct or through the health visitor who will investigate any difficulties that the parents are experiencing in bringing their child for examination and provide the necessary help, herself where possible or through the social services department of the relevant local authority.

6

The Vitreous and Aqueous Humour

The pressure of the eye is influenced by the pressure of the vitreous in the posterior segment of the eye and the aqueous filling the anterior chamber. Normally the vitreous volume remains constant (apart from vitreous loss caused by disease or severe trauma to the eye) and thus it is the aqueous which is mainly responsible for variations in intra-ocular pressure. Alteration in the rate of entry of aqueous into the eye from the ciliary processes, or in the rate of exit from the filtration angle, affects the intraocular pressure.

VITREOUS BODY

The vitreous body (or humour) is a semi-fluid, albuminous tissue which is transparent and which fills the space between the lens and the retina. It is hollowed out anteriorly for the reception of the lens and is surrounded by a hyaline membrane. If this membrance is disrupted by injury or operation displacement of the vitreous occurs.

The vitreous body fills the posterior four-fifths of the eye and maintains its shape. If, as a result of a perforating injury of the globe, vitreous escapes, the eye will shrink. It not only gives shape to the eye but maintains the retina in apposition to the choroid, so any loss of vitreous may predispose to retinal separation (see Chapter 5). If such a loss of vitreous occurs it cannot be replaced naturally but silicone, intravitreous air or normal saline may be used to make good the loss. The agent is introduced after retinal surgery to increase the pressure on the retina; after a few days air and normal saline are absorbed.

The vitreous has no blood supply but obtains its nourishment from the surrounding tissue.

In some people the vitreous is attached to the lens and in such cases a vitreous loss is inevitable during an intracapsular lens extraction (see p. 45). The jelly-like substance is easily recognized by a nurse watching such an operation or observing a patient with a severely damaged eye.

The vitreous becomes more fluid with advancing age, when shrinking may also occur.

Opacities of the vitreous are caused by the presence of remnants of blood vessels present in the eye during intrauterine development. The patient sees black threads or black spots which shift. Although these may worry an individual, reassurance can be given that they are not usually of any importance and are not likely to endanger sight, although occasionally floaters can be indicative of vitreous haemorrhage and may be the first warning of a detachment, so that the patient may be kept under review.

AQUEOUS HUMOUR

The aqueous is a fluid which is constantly produced by the capillary veins within the processes of the ciliary body. It passes from the posterior chamber through the pupil into the anterior chamber and leaves the eye through a sieve-like structure, the trabecula, at the drainage (filtration) angle. This is the angle formed by the root of the iris and the cornea.

From the trabecula the aqueous passes into the canal of Schlemm, a circular sinus at the junction of the cornea and the sclera which traverses the whole circumference of the eye, and then through a series of small aqueal vessels to the veins on the surface of the eye. A section of the anterior segment of the eye is shown in Fig. 28.

The drainage angle of the anterior chamber cannot be seen when looking at the eye because of its position within and behind the sclera.

To aid the ophthalmologist in viewing the drainage angle a special type of contact lens, known as a gonioscope (Fig. 29), has been developed. More detailed inspection of the area is possible with the combined use of the gonioscope and the slit-lamp microscope. Essentially this procedure involves the use of the slit-lamp beam which passes through the

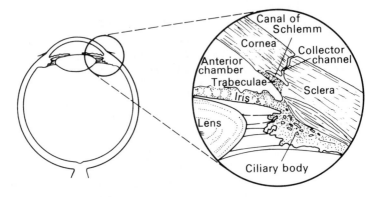

Fig. 28. *Section of the anterior segment of the eye, showing the anterior chamber, the trabeculae, the filtration angle, the canal of Schlemm and a collector channel*

special Goldmann lens in which is incorporated a mirror on to which the beam is directed. The effect of this is to deflect the image of the illuminated angle in the same direction of the objective lenses of the viewing microscope between which the light is centred.

INTRAOCULAR PRESSURE

Intraocular pressure is a measure of the amount of resistance of the sclera or cornea to compression. Normal intraocular pressure is between 18 and 24 mm of mercury, but there are variations of up to 3.5 mm in an individual during each 24 hours. The highest pressure usually occurs in the early hours of the morning during sleep.

Raised intraocular pressure may be periodic in its earlier stages but permanent when stenosis succeeds to spasm. After this any underlying systemic hypertension may worsen the damage which is caused in glaucoma by local ischaemia of the retina and of the optic nerve.

Digital Measurement

Measurement digitally, although not accurate, is useful as a quick reference to the state of the intraocular pressure, and with practice can easily be accomplished by the nurse.

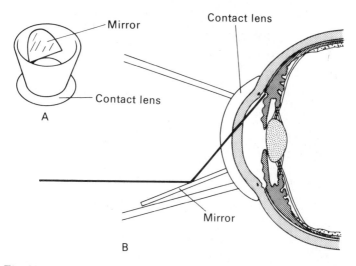

Fig. 29. *A, The Goldmann gonioscopic mirror. B, The mirror in use*

After seating the patient comfortably he is asked to look down. The nurse then gently palpates the eye through the upper lid using alternating pressure with her two index fingers (Fig. 30). This is repeated on the unaffected eye and a comparison made. The normal eye is said to feel like a 'ripe plum'. The pressure in early glaucoma is not sufficiently high to be detected by digital measurement.

An applanation tonometer is an even more precise instrument (Fig. 31), used with the slit-lamp microscope, which measures the pressure taken to flatten a small area of the cornea. For the use of this method the patient's full cooperation is essential to avoid any corneal damage and what is required of him must be explained carefully.

Tonographic measurement is a more elaborate form of tonometry using an electric tonometer which measures the outflow of aqueous. This involves holding a tonometer on the anaesthetized cornea for four minutes. Normally there should be a fall in the intraocular pressure as the weight of the tonometer forces the aqueous into the drainage

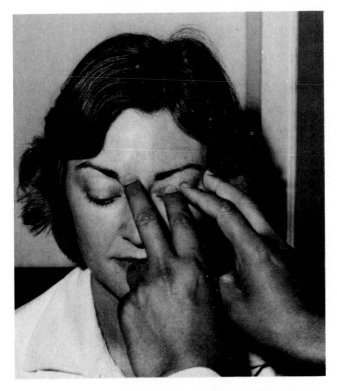

Fig. 30. *Testing the tension of the eyeball digitally*

angles; where the drainage of aqueous is inhibited, as in glaucoma, no drop in pressure occurs. A constant record is made in the form of a graph.

GLAUCOMA

Glaucoma is a condition in which the pressure within the eye is raised so that the visual field and sight are progressively destroyed.

Glaucoma may be classified according to the underlying causal abnormality:

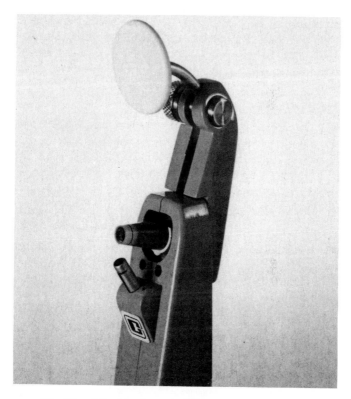

Fig. 31. *A Perkins hand-held applanation tonometer*

1. Closed-angle glaucoma, where the defect is one of narrowing of the drainage angle. This may be congenital.
2. Open-glaucoma where the defect is a progressive decrease in the permeability of the drainage meshwork (trabecula). This is essentially a disease of the middle aged or elderly.

CLOSED-ANGLE GLAUCOMA

In closed-angle glaucoma the eyes have a shallow anterior chamber so that the peripheral part of the iris lies very close to the drainage channels at the angle of the anterior chamber. A rise in pressure occurs when the iris comes into apposition with the cornea and closes the drainage channels. This leads to a sudden and acute rise in intraocular pressure to, for example, 50–60 mm mercury. A rise in intraocular pressure of this magnitude results in waterlogging of the cornea and cloudiness of vision.

There are two precipitating causes of angle closure:

1. *Pupillary block.* The root of the iris is thin and mobile and the pupil margin of the iris lies on the lens. Any slight increase in pressure of the aqueous behind it balloons the thin iris root forwards so that it comes into contact with the cornea, blocking the drainage channels.

2. *Any cause of pupil dilatation.* This occurs for example in darkness, on visiting the cinema, and is also induced by emotion and mydriatic drugs.

Subacute attacks of closed-angle glaucoma are transient episodes of blurring of vision, usually occurring in the evening. The patient complains of seeing 'haloes'—coloured rings round lights. These tend to be considered of little importance by the patient.

The nurse in the casualty department will be taught to recognize acute attacks immediately so that she may be able to anticipate the doctor's orders. The patient complains of severe pain, nausea and vomiting and of a rapid and severe reduction in vision. On examination by the doctor the eye will show ciliary injection; the cornea appears cloudy as a result of oedema and the anterior chamber is shallow. The pupil is fixed, semi-dilated and oval due to pressure of the sphincter of the iris. Digital palpation of the eye elicits a hard eye and quickly confirms the diagnosis (see p. 82) (Plate II/2).

Treatment

Glaucoma is an ophthalmic emergency and it must always be remembered that *total* loss of vision can occur if the pressure remains high for

24 hours. Some patients do not seek help for a number of days, thinking they have 'a cold in the eye', or sufferers from migraine may think they are experiencing another attack. Such patients will be in varying states of exhaustion requiring not only immediate treatment to the eye but also general nursing care.

Once the diagnosis has been made intensive treatment is begun, usually in the casualty department, to reduce the intraocular pressure. The first priority is to ensure the patient's comfort to enable him to cooperate in the rather lengthy treatment. He will appreciate being able to lie on a couch in a quiet area; explanation must be given of the treatment to be undertaken and the patient told of the possibility of admission to hospital. Any accompanying relatives or friends will also need to know how long the treatment will last to enable them to make any necessary arrangements.

The doctor will order various treatments to reduce the intraocular pressure. Pilocarpine 2% or 4% is used to constrict the pupil, draw the iris away from the cornea and open the drainage channels. This drug is short-lasting in action, compared with more powerful miotics and is relatively free from side effects. This treatment is carried out by the nurse and is known as intensive miotic treatment. It entails instilling the drops very frequently at first, and although time-consuming and tedious, it is a very necessary and effective measure. Variations in timing occur in different hospitals, but one regimen is:

1 drop every minute for 5 minutes
1 drop every 5 minutes for 15 minutes
1 drop every 15 minutes for 1 hour
1 drop every 30 minutes for 2 hours

To aid absorption of the drops, and for the general comfort of the patient, heat may be applied locally to the inflamed eye, the most convenient method being the electric heater (see Fig. 7).

Often there is found to be a less severe rise in the intraocular pressure of the apparently unaffected eye (from 25 to 30 mm mercury). Eye drops of pilocarpine 4% may be ordered to be instilled into this eye three times daily.

Acetazolamide may be prescribed. This drug inhibits the action of carbonic anhydrase, which is concerned in the transference of aqueous across the blood–aqueous barrier, and so reduces the production of aqueous through the ciliary processes. Acetazolamide is given initially in a dose of 500 mg by intravenous or intramuscular injection and then is continued by mouth at a dose of 250 mg six-hourly. Acetazolamide may occasionally give rise to paraethesia, renal colic or other unwanted effects, but in the absence of such side effects it can be given for long periods.

Of further benefit in the acute attack is the administration of such dehydrating and diuretic substances as oral glycerol, or intravenous infusions of mannitol or urea. The last two are sometimes given pre-operatively to reduce the intraocular pressure.

To control nausea an antiemetic preparation may be prescribed and in cases of severe pain morphine 10 mg may be required.

If this medical treatment reduces the pressure satisfactorily and the patient is sufficiently recovered he may be allowed to go home with miotic drops and acetazolamide tablets, careful explanation being given to him and to his relatives on how to carry out the regimen. He will be asked to return to the out-patient department for further investigations and follow up. However, after four hours intensive treatment a number of patients fail to respond sufficiently and hospital admission is necessary. Because of the severe pain and general physical disturbance the patient often readily accepts admission.

Preoperative Care

As the patient will be admitted as an emergency, preparations must be made quickly for his reception. The nurse will welcome him to the ward, help him to undress and get into bed and make him as comfortable as possible. Any accompanying relatives or friends are given the necessary information with regard to visiting and likely length of stay. If the patient has come alone, relatives should be notified at once, by telephone where possible, of his admission. The doctor will see the patient again and will probably order a second intensive course of miotic treatment with further intravenous or intramuscular acetazolamide.

The majority of patients respond to this second course of treatment, but for those who do not surgery is necessary. A peripheral iridectomy is performed to allow the free movement of aqueous from behind to in front of the iris. The uninvolved eye will also require a prophylactic peripheral iridectomy as the same predisposing anatomical configuration exists in this eye.

The surgical procedure is also often advisable in those patients who do not respond to out-patient medical treatment, as failure to continue the treatment, or an intervening illness which may cause them to forget the treatment may result in a sudden acute attack with further damage to the eye.

Postoperative Care

Postoperative care is similar to that of a patient who has undergone a lens extraction (see p. 47). After discharge from hospital regular visits are necessary to either a glaucoma or an ophthalmic clinic until the patient is maintaining a normal intraocular pressure.

OPEN-ANGLE GLAUCOMA

In this condition there is a moderate elevation of the intraocular pressure to 30 to 40 mm of mercury which, if untreated, leads to permanent damage to the eye. Pathological cupping of the optic disc occurs because this area is the weakest of all the intraocular structures and so gives way to pressure (Fig. 32). Visual field defects will follow as nerve fibres are destroyed by the cupping of the optic disc. This does not result directly in blindness, which may follow the subsequent nipping of the retinal blood vessels over the lip of the cupped disc causing ischaemia and death of retinal tissue.

Open-angle glaucoma is a progressive disease which affects the older age groups and is of insidious onset with *no symptoms* until the condition is well developed and damage to the optic nerve has already taken place. While the intraocular pressure is raised deterioration of vision is inevitable, and if unchecked may lead to blindness or at least to greatly reduced fields of vision.

The visual field refers to what can be seen with one eye closed, looking at a central spot (Fig. 33). Not only is there vision centrally but also at the sides, with some reduction on the side which is partially obstructed by the nose. An area of blindness in the visual field is referred to as a scotoma; in glaucoma this scotoma has a characteristic shape and is known as an arcuate scotoma.

Charting of the fields using a perimeter (Fig. 34) or Fieldman electronic scanner will reveal nerve destruction. Progress of the disease is measured by analysis of the tensions and by change in the visual field.

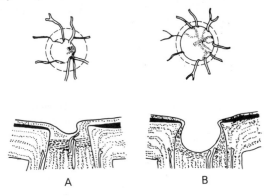

Fig. 32. *Cupping of the optic disc as seen on section of the nerve head and ophthalmoscopically. A, Physiological. B, Pathological*

Because of its slow, symptomless onset the early detection of open-angle glaucoma is very difficult, if not impossible, unless glaucoma surveys can be carried out. Since 2% of people over the age of 45 years are potential victims, ideally screening of all persons over this age should take place from time to time. Unfortunately most screening has been carried out only for research reasons and routine screening of the at-risk population is largely neglected. Usually the condition is detected on examination of the eyes by the presence of pathological cupping which indicates that the disease is already well advanced. The patient may complain of haloes round lights which result from the aqueous being pushed into the corneal substance giving him the impression that he is looking through rain drops.

Tests

Open-angle glaucoma is to a considerable extent hereditary in nature and provocative tests, that is tests to provoke a rise in tension when

PLATE I. The fundus

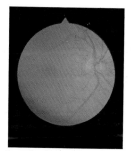

1. The normal fundus

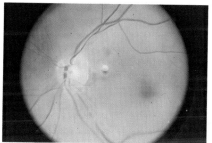

2. Occlusion of the central retinal artery

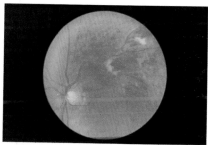

3. Thrombosis of a branch retinal vein

PLATE II. The 'red eye'

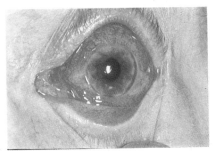

1. Acute closed angle glaucoma

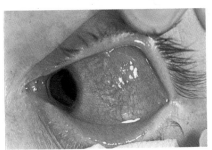

2. Acute follicular conjunctivitis

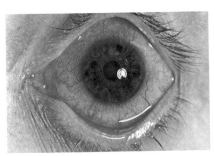

3. Iridocyclitis

the diagnosis is doubtful, may be carried out on marginal patients or near relatives of affected persons. Various tests are available.

Assessment of intraocular pressure As already stated there is a normal rise in intraocular tension in the early morning: in patients with glaucoma

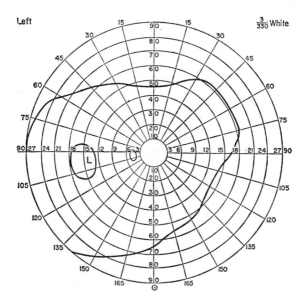

Fig. 33. *The normal peripheral vision of the left eye*

there may be a rise during the day also. Repeated tonometry at three-hourly intervals throughout the day and night will show if this is so.

Dark room test The normal dilatation of the pupil in the dark will cause some blockage of the drainage angle. This is especially true in closed-angle glaucoma. The pressure is recorded before and one hour after being in the dark room. The patient is not disturbed but is not allowed to sleep since there is a relaxation during sleep which would give a false reading. This must be explained to the patient to gain his cooperation. A transistor radio will help him to pass the time during the period in the dark room. A rise of tension of 5 mm of mercury or more is considered significant.

Water drinking test The patient drinks 1 litre of water within a period of five minutes. The tension is recorded before and at 15-minute intervals for one hour after drinking the water; if the tension has not

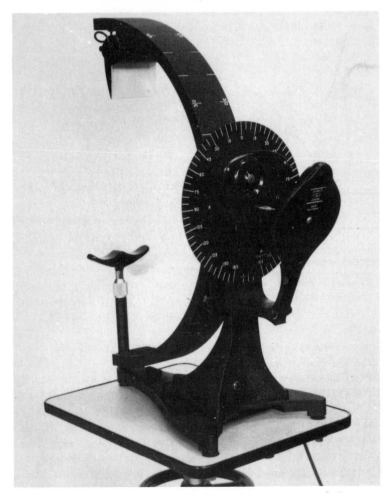

Fig. 34. *A Lister perimeter*

then returned to the original level the readings are continued. Ideally this test is carried out as an in-patient procedure. The patient should fast from midnight and the test be started early in the morning. One nurse should take all of the tonometry readings and record them. If the subject is an out-patient he must understand fully the preparation involved and the length of time he will be at the hospital. Again a rise in tension of 5 mm of mercury is significant, especially if it is associated with a slow return to the base line level.

Mydriatic test The tension of an eye with a normal pupil is compared with one with a dilated pupil. In an eye predisposed to glaucoma this tension may increase to above normal limits; a very mild mydriatic is used so that its effect can be reversed easily. If the test is carried out on an out-patient, he is not allowed home until miosis is achieved.

Treatment

Medical treatment for open-angle glaucoma is favoured in the first instance and continued as long as possible because of the frequent poor results obtained with surgery and the complications which attend the surgery itself.

Patients must be under regular supervision for measurement of the intraocular pressure and charting of the visual fields and so understanding and cooperation are essential. In all treatments which involve a complicated routine, especially when the treatment has to be carried out throughout the 24 hours, it may be necessary to consider admitting the patient to hospital, particularly if he is elderly. Inquiries should be made as to whether the patient lives alone or whether it would be possible to make arrangements for a relative or friend to stay with him during the period of treatment and supervise if necessary. The social conditions of the patient can be crucial to the success or failure of medical treatment.

Pilocarpine eye drops 2% or 4% are instilled at regular intervals throughout the 24 hours (eight-hourly or six-hourly). Pilocarpine is used to increase the outflow of aqueous by causing constriction of the ciliary body. Further control may be gained by the use of adrenaline eye drops 2% at night; these lower the resistance to the outflow of aqueous without causing constriction of the pupil. Constriction of the pupil is not always desirable in the elderly, especially when there are some lens changes, as it will cause visual impairment, particularly at night. Oral acetazolamide may be prescribed, but prolonged use is not desirable because of the possibility of the side effects already mentioned.

If medical therapy fails surgical drainage is performed: this consists of creating a new artificial exit of the aqueous from the eye which allows it to drain into the subchoroidal space. The operation is known as cyclodialysis. An iris inclusion, anterior flap sclerotomy or trabeculectomy allows the aqueous to drain externally through the subconjunctival tissues. These procedures are more accurate than both cyclodialysis and cyclodiathermy as it is difficult to control the effect of the latter two operations. If after surgery, there are repeated attacks and the eye is not suitable for further surgery, aqueous production may be reduced by external diathermy to the ciliary body (cyclodiathermy).

SECONDARY GLAUCOMA

Secondary glaucoma occurs when there is a rise in intraocular pressure resulting from an associated ocular disease, for example iritis or hypermature lens. It is important to prevent the onset of secondary glaucoma by treatment of the predisposing condition, but acetazolamide will be helpful in obtaining a temporary reduction in the intraocular pressure. Surgery may be necessary where medical methods fail.

STEROID GLAUCOMA

Steroid glaucoma occurs when raised intraocular pressure follows the use of topical steroids in a susceptible person; this usually subsides when the steroids are withdrawn or pilocarpine drops are used.

ABSOLUTE GLAUCOMA

An uncontrollable rise in intraocular pressure leading to a total loss of vision and pain is known as absolute glaucoma. This is treated either with a retrobulbar injection into the ciliary plexus of nerves of alcohol

60% to 90%, so rendering the eye painless, or by an enucleation of the eye.

THROMBOTIC GLAUCOMA

In cases of thrombosis of the central retinal vein, new vessels form on the iris which will slowly obliterate the filtration angle.

CONGENITAL GLAUCOMA (BUPHTHALMOS OR 'OX EYE')

Congenital glaucoma, present before birth, usually involves both eyes, though rarely equally. It is a familial disease which occurs when full development of the anterior chamber drainage angle has not taken place. As the intraocular pressure rises the eye stretches to accommodate the extra fluid.

Buphthalmos may not be apparent at birth, as, although the anatomical defects are congenital, the enlargement of the eyeball is not usually apparent until several months later. The condition is more common in males.

Since, in the first few months of life, the infant's closest companion and observer is his mother she may be the first to notice something amiss; on attending a general practitioner's well-baby clinic (or a local authority clinic) the mother may draw attention to signs of abnormal eye behaviour. The baby will then be referred to an ophthalmologist.

The nurse in an eye unit or hospital learns to pick out these children as they present such an unhappy face to the world with irritability and photophobia (sensitivity to light) as a result of corneal oedema. There is usually obvious enlargement of one or both eyes with an increased corneal diameter, greater than 12 mm; the normal value is up to 11 mm. The eyes appear large and saucer-like with haziness of the corneas caused by oedema, the aqueous having been pushed into the corneal tissues.

Preoperative Care

When the condition is discovered, early admission to hospital for assessment and operative treatment is usual.

The problems associated with the admission of babies and small children to hospital are discussed in the chapter dealing with retinoblastoma (see Chapter 5) and, although the prognosis in congenital glaucoma is not so serious, the same need exists for the mother to be admitted with her child where possible and other practical problems mentioned in the previous chapter apply equally here.

Consent for operation should be obtained from the parents and, after a thorough general examination, an examination of the eyes under a general anaesthetic is carried out. As the administration of a sedative may lower the intraocular pressure, intramuscular atropine 0.3–0.4 mg may be the only preoperative medication ordered for the child.

During the examination the corneal diameter is measured, the intraocular pressure recorded and an examination of the drainage angle carried out with a gonioscope. Miotic drops, which cause constriction of the sphincter of the pupil and thus increase the angle of drainage, may be prescribed. Miotics are used in the treatment of glaucoma as described below or to counteract the effects of mydriatics. Pilocarpine (0.5–4%) or eserine (0.125–1%) are the most commonly used miotics.

Operation

This takes the form of cutting the thickened tissue and the trabecula of the drainage angle thus making an opening (cleft) into the canal of Schlemm; this procedure is known as goniotomy. Other types of surgical treatment, as used in adult glaucoma, are not as a rule successful, as any drainage sinus quickly fills with new tissue, rendering the procedure useless.

Postoperative Care

After surgical treatment, miotic treatment is maintained and the child's condition reviewed at regular intervals. The role of the parents is most important as it will be necessary for them to continue to instil miotic drops after the child leaves hospital; indeed patients with glaucoma have to use these drops for the remainder of their lives. The interval between the instillation of the drops will depend upon the individual case, but the parents must realize that it is essential to instil them at the times prescribed. They should be warned that under this regimen the pupil will become very small and during the evening and in poor light the child's vision will be impaired. It should be understood that while miotics do not *cure* glaucoma their use will control intraocular pressure as long as treatment is maintained.

Before the child goes home the nurse should satisfy herself that his parents have grasped thoroughly how and when to instil the miotic drops prescribed and the importance of maintaining the treatment regularly.

The discovery, classification and care of all handicapped children is an important part of the school health service and a partially sighted child may require special schooling in order for him to fulfil his maximum educational potential. Here the hospital medical social worker, alerted by the doctor or by the nursing staff, will collaborate with the school medical officer so that the most suitable arrangements may be made. Wherever possible partially sighted children are taught in special day schools or in special classes in ordinary schools so that they may have as normal an education as possible.

Since congenital glaucoma is a familial condition, any other children in the family should be observed carefully for signs of the disease and often examination under anaesthesia is advised very early in life.

7

The Uveal Tract

The middle layer of the eyeball is made up of three separate but interconnected parts, the iris, the ciliary body and the choroid, which together are called the uveal tract or uvea.

Uveitis, or diseases of the component parts, may be endogenous, when the cause is generally unknown. Therefore it may be necessary to investigate the patient for a number of conditions including tuberculosis, sarcoidosis, syphilis, septic foci, allergy, virus disease, auto-immunity and metabolic upset. It is usually the case, however, that no specific cause can be found.

Cases can occasionally be traced to a perforating wound of the eyeball or corneal ulcers which may lead to extensive damage to the eye. These cases are in the minority.

IRIS

The iris is a coloured circular membrane situated behind the cornea and immediately in front of the lens; in the centre is an aperture, the pupil, which is variable in size (Fig. 35A). The margin of the pupil rests on the front portion of the lens capsule.

The iris partially divides the space containing the aqueous between the cornea and the lens into two parts, the anterior and posterior chambers.

The iris is attached at its periphery, or root, to the surface of the ciliary body; at this point it is relatively thin which explains why the iris may tear away from the ciliary body (iridodialysis) following an injury to the eye.

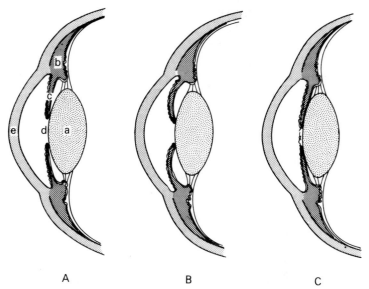

| A | B | C |

Fig. 35. *Anterior section of the eyeball. A, The normal iris.*
a = lens, b = ciliary body, c = iris, d = pupil, e = cornea.
B, Annular posterior synechia (occlusion of the pupil).
C, Total posterior synechia (occlusion of the pupil)

The structure of the iris consists of delicate connective tissue containing pigment cells, plain muscle, blood vessels and nerves.

The colour depends upon the arrangement of the iris pigment. In infancy the iris appears blue. This blueness may persist throughout life but usually pigment is deposited so that the iris assumes various colour patterns of green or brown.

MUSCLES

There are two sets of smooth muscle fibres, one arranged circularly so that on contraction there is narrowing of the pupil. These circular muscle fibres are excited by the action of light and contract, causing constriction of the pupil and shielding the retina from very bright light.

The fibres of the second set are arranged radially from the margin of the pupil and when contracted result in dilatation of the pupil. In dim light the radial muscle fibres are excited to contract and the pupil is thus dilated to permit the greatest amount of light to enter the eye.

The function of the iris is to regulate the amount of light entering the eye. Control of the muscles of the iris is exercised by the autonomic nervous system.

	Constriction	*Dilatation*
According to the amount of light	In bright light	In dim light
The effect of emotion	In anger	In fear
The action of drugs	Eserine, pilocarpine, morphine	Atropine

Constriction of the pupil also occurs during accommodation and in sleep.

INJURY

Hyphaema, blood in the anterior chamber, is a common condition seen in patients in the accident department of an eye hospital and is the result of an injury causing bleeding from the iris. This type of injury does not presuppose perforation of the eyeball, as a hyphaema may be caused by a blow such as that from a cricket ball.

Usually the blood is completely absorbed in a few days, although in some cases secondary bleeding may occur within a few hours or days of the original injury. For this reason the patient is admitted to hospital for rest and observation.

Complications which may follow an injury and hyphaema include:

1. Secondary glaucoma caused by blood blocking the filtration angle.
2. Iridodialysis. Here the iris is partially torn away from the ciliary body altering the shape of the pupil to a D-shape.
3. Commotio retinae. The retina becomes oedematous and, although the oedema subsides, pigment changes occur.

4. Traumatic mydriasis. The sphincter muscle of the iris becomes paralysed so that the pupil remains dilated and will not respond to light for several weeks following the injury.
5. Blood-staining of the endothelium of the cornea.

Treatment

The patient should be admitted to hospital. As he often feels fit he may not see any reason for this and may resist admission. A careful explanation should be given to him of the need for rest and observation of the condition of the eye in view of the possibility of any of the above complications taking place.

The patient should remain at rest in bed for four to seven days until the hyphaema has absorbed. He may, however, be taken to the lavatory in a chair at least once a day. Efforts should be made during this period of enforced rest to overcome the boredom which will be felt by an otherwise fit person. Once the hyphaema has absorbed, the patient is allowed gradually to become fully ambulant.

On admission antibiotic drops will have been instilled into the affected eye and a pad and bandage applied. The eye should be examined daily for secondary haemorrhage and for a rise in intraocular pressure. The former may require a paracentesis to allow the hyphaema to be evacuated: the latter should be treated by a carbonic anhydrase inhibitor such as acetazolamide.

Severe bruising of the lids may accompany the injury and the patient will need reassurance that the swelling and discoloration will subside.

Before the patient is discharged from hospital, a full examination of the fundus is undertaken to ascertain whether there are any retinal disturbances, for example retinal oedema, which would necessitate a longer stay in hospital until the condition had resolved. On discharge the patient will be advised to avoid any strenuous exercise or heavy lifting at least until he is seen again for a further examination two weeks after discharge.

Albinism is a hereditary condition in which there is a marked deficiency of pigment in the body; the subject has white hair and eyelashes and the iris lacks pigment. There is intense photophobia and nystagmus and myopic changes are present. Good vision is usually possible with the aid of the correct tinted spectacles to overcome the visual defect.

CILIARY BODY

The ciliary body connects the choroid with the circumference of the iris. It is arranged in folds radiating inwards which comprise the ciliary processes surrounding the margin of the lens. These processes are well supplied with blood vessels and nerves; they produce aqueous by a process of dialysis and secretion. The ciliary muscle fibres arise from the sclera and extending backwards are inserted into the ciliary processes. This muscle is used in the process of accommodation and affects the convexity of the lens.

CHOROID

The brown membrane lining the inner surface of the sclera is the choroid; it contains many blood vessels and pigment cells which render it dark and opaque. The choroid is separated from the sclera by a lymph space but is attached to it by connective tissue. The choroid supplies nutrients to the retina and vitreous and also serves to prevent internal reflection of light.

The most common condition which affects the uveal tract is uveitis. This can be divided into anterior uveitis, or iridocyclitis, and posterior uveitis, or choroiditis. Iridocyclitis is not uncommon and if left untreated may lead to blindness or result in serious complications such as secondary glaucoma.

The blood vessels around the limbus become dilated and give rise to ciliary injection, an important sign which nurses must not confuse with conjunctival injection (see p. 119) (Plate II/3).

The pupil is small and if a mydriatic drop is instilled will dilate irregularly. This is the result of adhesions between the margin of the iris and the underlying lens capsule. If the eye is left untreated, the pupillary margin may become completely adherent to the lens giving rise to the condition of iris bombé (Fig. 35B) in which there is an increase in the intraocular pressure as the aqueous is unable to pass from the posterior to the anterior chamber. White blood cells accumulate in the anterior chamber and may clump together on the posterior surface of the cornea; these may be seen with the aid of the slit lamp and are called keratic precipitates (KP). In very severe cases pus forms at the base of the anterior chamber—hypopyon.

Many cases of anterior uveitis are the result of a systemic disease; two examples are collagen diseases and diabetes mellitus. Focal streptococcal infections of the teeth, tonsils and sinuses can also be a causative factor.

Treatment

It is important that patients with anterior uveitis should undergo a thorough physical examination and any necessary investigations in order to detect any possible underlying disease for which referral for specialized medical treatment will be required. Local treatment must be begun as soon as possible.

Long-acting mydriatic drops are instilled to dilate the pupil and to break down the adhesions of the iris to the lens (posterior synechia (Fig. 35B, C). If this treatment does not prove effective a subconjunctival injection of a mydriatic may be necessary (see p. 28).

Steroid drops are also instilled in order to reduce the inflammatory processes and prevent complications; if necessary steroids may also be given by subconjunctival injection. Systemic steroids may be given to some patients. Local heat in the form of hot bathes may be comforting and dark glasses are worn to relieve the photophobia, which can be distressing.

Very severe cases will necessitate admission to hospital in order to ensure regular treatment. Patients who are debilitated or living in difficult social conditions will benefit from a period of rest in bed, general nursing care and attention to diet.

CHOROIDITIS

Choroiditis (posterior uveitis) is less obvious on visual examination and is diagnosed on ophthalmoscopic examination. The patient usually complains of hazy vision which is the result of exudation from the choroid passing into the vitreous. Choroiditis may be present as part of a generalized uveitis when the signs of anterior uveitis may also be seen.

Swelling of the choroid may cause interruption to the nourishment of the retina which may lead to retinal separation.

The local treatment is as for anterior uveitis but for this condition also it may be necessary to give systemic steroids, as the use of local applications is of limited value. Here again investigation of the general health of the patient is important; tuberculosis may be the underlying cause of the condition.

TOXOPLASMOSIS

Toxoplasmosis is a protozoal infestation which may be congenital or acquired. This infection is common in rodents, birds and dogs. The condition affects the retina and choroid of both eyes and may also affect other systems of the body. Young children admitted to hospital suffering from apparent blindness may in fact have this condition which is sometimes associated with meningeal changes. Treatment is by the administration of antimalarial drugs.

SARCOIDOSIS

The cause of sarcoidosis is unknown; it often closely resembles tuberculosis. It may affect the eyes, producing primarily a granulomatous uveitis. There may be nodules in the iris and profuse keratic precipitates, but only occasionally choroidal involvement. The uveitis runs a chronic, prolonged course with occasional acute flare-ups and may lead to secondary glaucoma, cataract or phthisis bulbi, so that after a time the eye may be damaged beyond repair. There is no specific treatment but cortisone or ACTH may be ordered to inhibit the inflammatory response in acute phases in the absence of any secondary infection.

TUMOURS OF THE UVEAL TRACT

A melanoma of the iris or ciliary body may develop and can be removed surgically together with an area of healthy tissue. If the choroid is involved an enucleation of the eye is necessary.

8

The Cornea and Sclera

THE CORNEA

The cornea is the transparent avascular tissue which forms the anterior one-sixth of the eyeball and is about 11 mm in diameter. It is continuous with but thicker than the sclera. The point at which the cornea and sclera meet is known as the corneoscleral junction or limbus. In the elderly, fatty degeneration may cause a white ring known as arcus senilis (Fig. 36) to form at the limbus; this develops gradually until the ring is complete. No treatment is needed as the condition is symptom-free and the transparency of the central cornea is not affected.

The cornea is composed of five layers of tissue: the epithelium, Bowman's membrane, stroma, Descemet's membrane and endothelium (Fig. 37). The epithelium on the outer surface is continuous with the conjunctiva; any damage to this layer heals readily. Normal corneal epithelium is very sensitive to touch, and thus has a protective function. Some long-standing conditions affecting the cornea, for example a dendritic ulcer (see. p. 107), may render it insensitive. Any damage to Bowman's membrane, which lies beneath the epithelium, will heal with scar formation. The thickest part of the corneal structure is the stroma, a transparent fibrous connective tissue which comprises 90% of the cornea. Below the stroma is a thin, firm but highly elastic layer called Descemet's membrane. The deepest layer, the endothelium, is a row of cells which play a part in controlling the amount of fluid in the cornea. Nourishment of the cornea is achieved through the aqueous in contact with the deepest layers, and the tears on the outer surface.

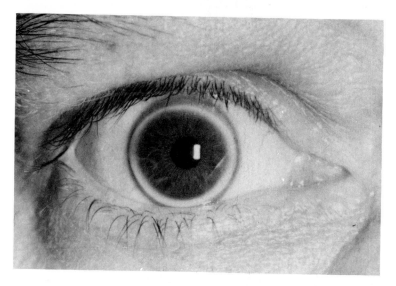

Fig. 36. *Arcus senilis*

The exposed position of the cornea is the principal reason why it is vulnerable to pathology by accidental trauma and ulceration. Some of the conditions that may affect the cornea are dealt with.

KERATITIS

Inflammation of the cornea, keratitis, is a common condition conveniently divided into two types:

1. Ulcerative keratitis, often known as corneal ulceration, in which there is some destruction of a portion of the epithelium.
2. Non-ulcerative keratitis, in which, although all the layers of the cornea are affected by the inflammatory process, the epithelium remains intact.

Symptoms

Photophobia is the most characteristic symptom of keratitis; pain and lacrimation are also present. There is defective vision as the normal transparency and curvature of the cornea is affected by the inflammatory

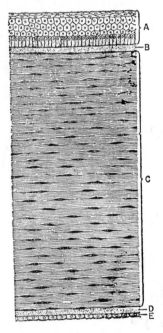

Fig. 37. *The histological appearance of the cornea. A, Epithelium. B, Bowman's membrane. C, Stroma. D, Descemet's membrane. E, Endothelium*

process. When ulceration occurs a pit is formed on the corneal surface; this can be readily demonstrated as the tissue, denuded of epithelium on the ulcerated area, will stain green when a drop of fluorescein 2% is instilled. If the epithelium alone is damaged, the ulcer will heal in a few days without scarring, but if the ulcer has penetrated into the stroma of the cornea a scar which will result in an opacity will form. A fine, small scar is termed a nebula and a large, dense scar a leucoma. When an ulcer is particularly deep a collection of inflammatory cells form a solid yellow mass in the lower part of the anterior chamber: this is known as hypopyon (pus in the anterior chamber). In a few instances the pus may completely fill the anterior chamber.

ULCERATIVE KERATITIS

Corneal Ulceration (Secondary to Conjunctivitis)

In staphylococcal, pneumococcal or streptococcal conjunctivitis small marginal corneal ulcers may form. These cause considerable pain, photophobia and blepharospasm (spasm of the eyelids). The ulcers usually heal quickly as the conjunctivitis subsides. In treating conjunctivitis, a swab should be taken to determine the causative organism and the drugs to which it is sensitive, and the appropriate antibiotic drops or ointment instilled.

Herpetic Ulceration

Ulceration caused by the herpes simplex virus is becoming more common. The herpetic corneal ulceration is often associated with a herpetic vesicle of the facial skin, most commonly around the lips (commonly known as a 'cold sore') or on the side of the face. A distinctive form of this type of keratitis is the dendritic ulcer; this ulcer resembles the branching of a tree (dendron) and spreads superficially over the cornea. The inflammatory process encourages the entry of blood vessels into the cornea which in turn leads to scarring.

Treatment Local treatment aims to destroy the virus before the deep corneal tissue is involved. The use of IDU (5 iodo-2-deoxyuridine) drops, an antiviral agent, may eliminate the need to cauterize the cornea if the treatment is carried out in the early stages of the condition. To be effective drops must be instilled frequently (one- to two-hourly) throughout the 24 hours for several days. It may be necessary to admit the patient to hospital for this intensive treatment. Mydriatic drops may also be used to dilate the pupil. Topical steroid drops are contraindicated in the presence of active infection as they enhance viral replication. However, they are sometimes used in disciform keratitis to help prevent vascularization when no active epithelial lesion is present.

The application of cryotherapy has been used to prevent the spread of lesions with promising results. An attempt should be made to find any contributory causative lesions; any such lesions being treated appropriately.

If the ulceration does not respond to treatment a central tarsorrhaphy may be necessary. In this operation the centres of the two lid margins are sutured together to keep the lids closed; a deep mattress-type suture is inserted and small rubber tubes threaded through the suture and placed next to the skin surface of the lids. Eye drops can be instilled at the sides where the lid margins are not sutured. The sutures and rubber tubes can be removed after 10–14 days as by this time the lids will have become adherent and can remain so until separated by cutting with sharp scissors. There should be no residual scarring of the lids; the eyelashes will remain intact.

Exposure Keratitis

Exposure keratitis may be due to some deformity of the lids, caused by trauma, paralysis of the facial nerve or severe exophthalmos. Fine, slightly depressed areas appear on the corneal surfaces and are known as punctate epithelial erosions. The treatment will depend upon the cause.

Mooren's Ulcer

A chronic, painful, indolent ulcer, Mooren's ulcer, occurs in the absence of any obvious infection. It is usually seen in elderly people and both eyes may be involved. The ulcer begins near the upper margin of the cornea and spreads gradually; whilst one part of the ulcer is healing the other is advancing.

Treatment is not very satisfactory. Keratoplasty (corneal grafting) does not bring about a cure as the donor cornea is liable to be affected by a spread of the disease from the host cornea. Beta irradiation is a more effective treatment and may be undertaken in the out-patient department.

NON-ULCERATIVE KERATITIS

Interstitial Keratitis

With a deep interstitial keratitis there is opacity of the stroma of the cornea and no ulceration but some signs of uveitis. Usually one eye only is involved, with a severe loss of vision. The condition is associated with a number of diseases, for example, syphilis, tuberculosis, lupus erythematosus and leprosy. In children the condition may result from congenital syphilis when the second eye may be attacked although perhaps not for weeks or months later. However, congenital syphilis is rarely seen today owing to good antenatal care of the mother.

Treatment will be given to the underlying cause. Topical steroids reduce corneal damage. Mydriatic drops are used when there is involvement of the uveal tract, dilatation of the pupil avoiding the formation of synechia and resting the eye by paralysing the ciliary muscles.

Disciform Keratitis

Disciform keratitis also occurs in the stroma of the cornea, a grey, disc-shaped opacity developing. It may be the result of a viral infection entering through a small defect in the cornea and commonly follows herpes of the cornea. Topical steroids are indicated in the treatment of disciform keratitis.

KERATOPLASTY

Corneal grafting, keratoplasty, was first carried out in England in the 1930s. Its aim is to replace a scarred cornea, or part of a cornea, with a healthy one. The prognosis will depend to a large extent upon the underlying cause of the scarring.

Occasionally, if the patient has one eye with a healthy cornea but a diseased retina and the other eye with corneal scarring, it may be desirable to graft the healthy cornea on to the other eye. In this case good results can be expected as the possibility of rejection by immunological reaction will not occur.

In most cases the donor cornea comes from another individual and some reaction may take place resulting in corneal opacity. However, corneal grafts are one of the most successful forms of transplantation and the use of steroids has helped to overcome the problem of rejection.

There are two forms of keratoplasty:

1. Lamellar keratoplasty, when a superficial scar is removed and replaced by a half thickness graft.
2. Full-thickness or penetrating keratoplasty in which the total scarred area is removed and replaced with a full thickness graft. This type of graft involves opening the eyeball with the possible risk of introducing infection and the problem of unity and healing of the round edges since the graft must heal with its edges exactly flush with the surrounding cornea.

In the past the average stay in hospital for a patient who had undergone a full thickness keratoplasty was between six and eight weeks, but with the introduction of microsurgery, fine suturing material and atraumatic needles and the development of surgical instruments, the in-patient period has been reduced to as little as one to two weeks.

Donor Eyes

The Human Tissue Act of 1953 allows an individual to bequeath his eyes for the purpose of corneal grafting, but eyes which are to be used for this purpose must be removed within 12 hours of the death of the donor. The eye is refrigerated at a temperature of 4°C. Eyes to be used for a full-thickness graft must be used within four days and those for a lamellar graft within seven days. The donor eyes must be free from corneal disease and glaucoma. The eyes are prepared in various ways and the nurse will need to become familiar with the method in use in the hospital in which she is working.

Eye banks have now become established in all major cities in England and research is still being undertaken into the methods of freezing tissue to make better use of the cornea available.

Nurses may be asked by patients or their relatives how to donate their eyes to an eye bank after death. Some hospitals have a leaflet giving information on the subject, otherwise it would be best for the nurse to advise inquirers to write to the Royal National Institute for the Blind (RNIB), whose headquarters are at 224 Great Portland Street, London W1, for information.

Preoperative Care

The patient is admitted to hospital 48 hours before operation for the necessary investigations. This will give him time to settle down in the ward and become familiar with his surroundings, the nursing staff and his fellow patients. It is particularly important that the patient understands that if suitable donor material is not available the operation may have to be postponed. This will inevitably cause disappointment and anxiety as the patient may have had corneal opacities for a long time and will have prepared himself psychologically for the operation which he hopes is going to restore his sight. The nurse must have a sympathetic understanding of the extent of the feelings of disappointment and frustration that a patient may feel in such an event. She must know that he will also be worried about how long it is likely to be before he can again be admitted for keratoplasty.

The local preoperative care usually includes the taking of a conjunctival swab for culture and sensitivity test (see p. 18); the lacrimal sacs are syringed (see p. 23) and the lashes of the eye to be operated on are cut (see p. 22). Antibiotic eye drops are instilled six-hourly until the time of operation. On the evening before the operation, and in the morning, miotic drops are also instilled to constrict the pupil and avoid lens damage if the operation is to be a penetrating keratoplasty.

The operation is carried out under general anaesthesia as it may be very long.

The Operation

The operation can be described in three stages:

1. The preparation of the donor material. When a lamellar keratoplasty is to be performed, this may be done after the scarred area of the host cornea has been removed as the surgeon is then better able to estimate the amount of donor material required and prepare it.

2. The removal of the diseased cornea. This is done either by the careful 'shaving off' of the diseased area in preparation for a lamellar keratoplasty or by using a trephine to remove the full thickness of the cornea for a penetrating keratoplasty.
3. The suturing of the donor material in position.

Postoperative Care

When the patient has recovered from the anaesthetic, and unless there are instructions to the contrary, he may be made comfortable in the semirecumbent position with two or three pillows. Some surgeons prefer their patients to have both eyes padded for the first 24—48 hours. If this is so, the patient will feel very confused and perhaps frightened. It should have been explained to him before the operation that both eyes may be covered and it is particularly important that after the operation the nurse takes time to explain fully what is being done for him on all occasions.

The nursing care for this patient is as for the patient who has undergone a lens extraction (see p. 47).

The first dressing is carried out under the supervision of the surgeon. Before beginning the blinds in the ward should be drawn as bright light will cause the patient distress. After explanation of the procedure, the prepared trolley is brought to the bedside. When the outer bandage has been removed, adhesive material holding the pad in position is cut and the pad removed. The lids should be swabbed carefully and the eye opened gently; an anaesthetic drop may be instilled to lessen the pain and discomfort caused by the presence of the sutures which may make the patient squeeze his eyelids.

The eye is then carefully inspected, particular note being taken of the depth of the anterior chamber, the position of the graft and whether there is any corneal oedema. A conjunctival swab may be taken. Mydriatic drops are instilled so that the pupil becomes widely dilated, as this will avoid adhesions forming between the iris and the wound. At the same time antibiotic drops will be instilled.

After the first dressing the patient is usually left with only the affected eye padded. He is then gradually mobilized and should be fully ambulant between the fourth and eighth days. By this time he will be permitted to wear dark glasses. Quite frequently a patient will complain that his eye is watering. This excess lacrimation is caused by the corneal sutures which act as an irritant. If this is explained to the patient it will dispel any fears that he may have.

Occasionally small blood vessels grow into the grafted area from the surrounding host cornea, and steroid drops may be used to halt their advance. Oedema of the graft may occur and is an early sign of rejection, but the use of systemic steroids helps to overcome this.

When the patient is discharged from hospital at the end of one or two weeks, he must be given very careful instructions concerning the instillation of drops in order to avoid damage to the grafted area. He should be advised to return to the clinic if he is at all worried about his eyes. Subsequently he will attend regularly at two- or three-weekly intervals until complete healing has taken place and the corneal sutures can be removed. This is carried out after the instillation of anaesthetic drops and with the patient seated at a slit-lamp.

CORNEAL INJURY

Much can be done by way of precautions and education of the public to prevent the occurrence of corneal injuries. Protective goggles and other safety devices must be available where workers are likely to sustain eye injuries and they must be taught to wear them properly and at all times when at risk. Fireworks carelessly handled are a likely source of corneal injury, and it is important that parents and children should be taught how to avoid this danger.

When foreign bodies enter the eye some will be found loose in the conjunctival sac or under the upper lid, but most are retained on the surface of the cornea. If they are not removed before the end of two or three days keratitis will develop. Some foreign bodies are very difficult to see and good illumination with a slit-lamp is needed.

A nurse in an accident department will deal with many patients who complain of 'something in my eye'. It is very important that a careful examination is undertaken of each eye.

Surface foreign bodies are very easily removed. The patient is seated in a chair and an anaesthetic drop instilled into the affected eye. The foreign body is located and lifted off the cornea with a fine pointed needle, for example a Saunders' needle. The small abraded area that is left is treated by the instillation of mydriatic and antibiotic drops and the eye covered with a pad and bandage. The patient is asked to return to the clinic daily for treatment until healing has taken place. This can be demonstrated by the instillation of fluorescein drops which will leave no green stain when the area is healed.

Deep foreign bodies may penetrate through to the stroma of the cornea and since removal may cause unjustifiable damage they may be left.

There are a few cases when the foreign body perforates the cornea and enters the anterior chamber, causing a loss of aqueous. Patients suffering this injury must be admitted to hospital at once in order to have the foreign body removed surgically and the perforation sutured.

INTRAOCULAR FOREIGN BODIES

When foreign bodies enter the eye at speed the patient often experiences little more than a twinge of pain. This type of accident may occur when a person is using a hammer and chisel; a small fragment of metal breaks off with sufficient momentum to enter the eye. Because of its exposed situation, the cornea is the most common site of entry of such a foreign body.

A large intraocular foreign body will cause such damage as to warrant immediate admission to hospital for surgical removal and repair. The entrance will be visible and often a piece of iris forms a plug in the wound. Small foreign bodies may cause less obvious signs. Very careful examination is essential.

In both cases radiographic examinations are necessary to detect the intraocular foreign body and find its position accurately.

Early detection and removal of an intraocular foreign body will increase the possibility of some sight being retained in the affected eye. If a copper or iron foreign body is left in the eye chemical reactions may take place. Many intraocular foreign bodies are of magnetic material and techniques are available to remove these with the aid of a magnet.

Corneal injuries may be so severe that the damaged tissue must all be removed and the wound sutured. The result of this treatment may be either a useless eye which is comfortable or one that is painful and may constitute a danger to the other eye. Then it must be removed (see sympathetic ophthalmia, p. 116).

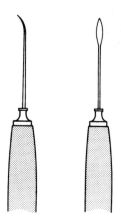

Fig. 38. *Saunders' needle for the removal of a corneal foreign body*

Simple perforating wounds are sutured, the prolapsed iris abscised and the anterior chamber reformed.

Preoperative Care

A patient with severe corneal injuries will be admitted to the ward from the accident department as an emergency. He will be prepared for operation with the minimum of delay. The patient, whether adult or child, who has suffered such an accident will be shocked and frightened and may be very confused at this stage.

Postoperative Care

It is usually in the immediate postoperative period that the patient will be most disturbed and anxious over the possibility of losing his sight and will need a great deal of support, reassurance and explanation from the nursing staff. If the injury is severe the surgeon will have warned the patient, or the parents of a child, of the possible outcome.

Patients who have had repair of severe injuries are kept at rest in bed for several days. This allows blood in the anterior chamber to be absorbed and healing of the wound to take place. It may be necessary for the patient to be fed and bathed by the nurse and at these times he may reveal to her his fear and anxiety concerning the possible loss of an eye. It is important that the doctor talks to the patient about the future and, if an enucleation is likely to be necessary, the implications of this should be clearly and simply explained. The nurse should reinforce what the doctor has said and allow the patient to express his feelings, at the same time helping him to adjust to the prospect of being left with only one eye. She may discuss with him the fitting of an artificial eye and it will be of help if she can arrange for a person who has overcome this situation to talk to the patient.

SYMPATHETIC OPHTHALMIA

A complication which may occur after a perforating injury is sympathetic ophthalmia, particularly if there is involvement of the ciliary body. The exact nature of the condition is not known, but an allergic response in the injured eye excites a reaction in the uninjured which is then called the sympathizing eye.

A uveitis develops in the uninjured eye and the usual treatment is to remove the injured eye. Occasionally, however, the injured eye is retained if it is thought there is likely to be more vision in that eye than in the uninjured one.

THE SCLERA

The sclera is easily recognized as the 'white' of the eye and forms five-sixths of the protective outer coat; the cornea forms the remaining one-sixth anteriorly. In structure the sclera is composed of firm, un-yielding fibrous tissue almost 1 mm thick; it is white on the outside, the internal surface is pale brown in appearance.

The outer surface of the sclera is covered by loose vascular tissue, the episcleral tissue, which is separated from the overlying conjunctiva by a thin layer of more dense fibrous tissue, Tenon's capsule. These structures can easily be seen by the nurse in the living eye when watching operations for the correction of strabismus (squint). At the junction of the cornea and the sclera is a continuous sinus, the canal of Schlemm; the aqueous from the anterior chamber drains into this canal.

In children the sclera may have a blue tinge because it is thin and the underlying pigmented choroid shows through. In old age deposits of fat may give the sclera a yellow appearance. The strong and inelastic tissue of which the sclera is composed maintains the shape of the eyeball and affords protection to the delicate structures within.

There are few conditions which affect the sclera:

1. *Scleritis.* Inflammation of the sclera in which the blood vessels tend to appear purplish in colour.
2. *Episcleritis.* Inflammation of a localized area of the episcleral tissue. The area appears red and may be swollen and painful.

Both these conditions are collagen diseases and thus may be associated with rheumatism or arthritis. Treatment is by the administration of topical steroids.

3. *Staphyloma.* An area of thinned sclera which bulges outwards with the underlying uveal tissue. It is a condition which may follow long periods of glaucoma or which may occur in persons with severe myopia.

Injury to the sclera may occur either as a result of a metal fragment entering the eye at speed and penetrating to become an intraocular foreign body, or with accidents with sharp instruments such as scissors. As these injuries are usually associated with cornea damage, the reader is referred to the section dealing with corneal injuries (pp. 113—114).

9

The Conjunctiva

The conjunctiva is a mucous membrane which lines the eyelids and is reflected on to the eyeball to cover it anteriorly as far as the limbus, where it merges into the superficial layer of the cornea.

The conjunctiva lining the eyelids, the palpebral conjunctiva, is highly vascular and through it can be seen the meibomian glands—the sebaceous glands at the edge of the eyelids. It is thicker than the bulbar conjunctiva covering the eyeball to the corneal margin. The sclera is visible through the bulbar conjunctiva.

The palpebral and bulbar conjunctiva are separated by a potential space, the conjunctival sac, which is formed by the reflection of the conjunctiva over the under-surface of the lids and the scleral section. There is a small red fleshy body, the caruncle, lying at the inner corner of the eye which becomes isolated during development.

The conjunctiva forms a protection for the underlying sclera and provides moisture to the eye by means of mucous and serous glands. The palpebral artery supplies the skin of the lids and the ophthalmic and facial arteries supply the whole of the eyelids and the conjunctiva. Whilst the conjunctiva is well supplied with blood vessels these are normally constricted and scarcely visible. Conjunctival injection or dilatation of these vessels occurs for various reasons and is termed conjunctivitis.

CONJUNCTIVITIS

Inflammation of the conjunctiva, known as red or pink eye, is very common. A red eye may be a sign of any one of several eye conditions; it is important that the correct diagnosis is made and appropriate treatment given. In patients with an inflamed eye caused by acute glaucoma prompt treatment may prevent loss of sight. The three most common causes of a red eye are all seen by nurses working in the casualty department and their differential diagnosis is outlined in the table below; they are illustrated in Plate II.

	Acute Conjunctivitis	*Acute Iritis*	*Acute Glaucoma*
Pain	'Grittiness'	Moderate	Severe
Discharge	May be purulent	Slight epiphora	Slight epiphora
Pupil	Normal	Constricted and fixed later irregular	Dilated, oval and fixed
Iris	Normal	'Muddy'	Greenish hue
Tension	Normal	Normal	Very hard

Patients who present in the casualty department with the signs and symptoms of conjunctivitis have a discharge which is often purulent. For the most effective use of antibiotics, it is desirable to obtain a conjunctival swab (see p. 18) for culture and sensitivity testing of the infecting organism, although routine treatment with a wide spectrum drug will normally be instituted immediately.

An infected eye with a discharge but normal vision suggests some form of conjunctivitis. The patient usually complains of discomfort with a gritty feeling in his eye and photophobia.

Conjunctivitis is usually the result of an infection—bacterial, fungal or viral. It may be acute, subacute or chronic. In some instances the condition may be an allergic response and occasionally is related to such skin disorders as rosacea.

The discharge is watery when the conjunctivitis is caused by a foreign body or an allergic or viral infection, but is mucopurulent in the presence of a bacterial or fungal infection.

ACUTE OR SUBACUTE INFECTIVE CONJUNCTIVITIS

Usually both eyes are affected simultaneously or infection of one eye may be followed shortly by spread to the other in infective conjunctivitis. In the case of young infants it is helpful to advise the mother to lay the baby on the side of the affected eye so that any discharge may not run across the nose to infect the other eye.

The lids are sticky, particularly on waking in the morning, and there may be excoriation of the lid margins. It has already been said that the condition may be caused by a number of organisms; it is contagious and outbreaks of 'pink eye' may occur where conditions are overcrowded and standards of hygiene low.

The degree of redness of the eye varies according to the nature and severity of the infection. It is less intense in the circumcorneal region, in contrast to the ciliary injection associated with acute iritis and glaucoma. In severe cases there may be chemosis in which the conjunctiva is swollen.

Treatment

The patient with conjunctivitis is usually treated in the out-patient department; appropriate anti-infective eye drops are prescribed for regular administration during the day and ointment at night. The use of ointment will help to reduce the stickiness of the lids in the morning. If the patient is treated as an out-patient, the regimen must be strictly adhered to and the patient will need specific instruction and demonstration.

Parents of children and adults suffering from bacterial conjunctivitis must understand the importance of using individual face flannels and towels to avoid the possible spread of the infection to other members of the family. Tissues should be used in place of handkerchiefs and should be disposed of after being used *once only*.

Some relief of discomfort can be obtained by removing any crusting from the lids by gentle swabbing with saline, each swab being used once only and then discarded. Photophobia can be overcome by wearing dark glasses. The use of a celluloid shade over the infected eye is to be condemned as it provides a favourable environment for the multiplication of micro-organisms.

OPHTHALMIA NEONATORUM

Gonococcal infection of the eyes of neonates is caused by direct infection during the passage down the birth canal in a mother suffering from gonorrhoea. This severe bilateral conjunctivitis is termed

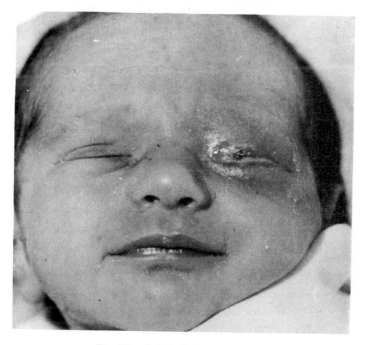

Fig. 39. *Ophthalmia neonatorum*

ophthalmia neonatorum (Fig. 39). Other organisms may also give rise to this condition but with less severe results. All cases of ophthalmia neonatorum beginning within 21 days of birth must be notified to the environmental health officer of the local authority.

Treatment

The treatment of ophthalmia neonatorum demands a special mention as in this condition large amounts of purulent secretion accumulate under tension under the tightly closed, swollen lids. Care must be taken when the lids are parted by nurse or doctor as this infective material could spurt up into their faces.

In severe cases there is rapid involvement of the cornea which may result in perforation and infection of the whole eye (panophthalmitis) with a subsequent shrinkage of the eye (phthisis bulbi).

In some maternity units prophylactic measures are carried out routinely on the newborn. The eyelids are swabbed and 10% sulphacetamide drops instilled into both eyes.

VIRAL CONJUNCTIVITIS

Viral conjunctivitis is usually accompanied by the formation of follicles and the condition is therefore also known as follicular conjunctivitis; however, allergic reactions may also result in the formation of follicles and it must not be assumed that a virus is always the cause of this type of conjunctivitis (Plate II/2).

There are several different forms of viral conjunctivitis which include:

1. *Inclusion* or 'swimming bath' conjunctivitis caused by one of the TRIC viruses and having an incubation period of five to nine days. Treatment is similar to that for bacterial types of conjunctivitis but response is often less satisfactory and relapses may occur.
2. *Trachoma.* This is discussed on p. 158.
3. *Reiter's syndrome* is a general medical condition in which a mild conjunctivitis, usually bilateral, is associated with non-specific urethritis, polyarthritis and pyrexia. The condition is usually seen in young men.

CHRONIC CONJUNCTIVITIS

Chronic conjunctivitis may follow either acute or repeated attacks or may be associated with the excessive use of local drugs. In some patients it is caused by undue exposure of the bulbar conjunctiva, as in exophthalmic goitre, proptosis or ectropion or where there is defective drainage of tears through the lacrimal passages. The patient complains of 'eye strain' and a sensation of grittiness and heat. Relief of the symptoms may be achieved by the application of local steroids.

ALLERGIC CONJUNCTIVITIS

Allergic conjunctivitis is seen usually in the spring and summer and results from exposure to allergens such as pollen. The patient will complain of discomfort and intense irritation. Flattened papillae form on the conjunctiva and the cornea may become involved. Allergic conjunctivitis may occur in association with other allergic reactions such as asthma and hay fever.

Treatment consists of the instillation of steroid eye drops, though for a few patients systemic steroid therapy may be required. In some instances the condition is so disabling that the papillae are removed and the conjunctiva replaced with a mucosal graft, the donor area being the inner surface of the mouth.

SUBCONJUNCTIVAL HAEMORRHAGE

Subconjunctival haemorrhage is often caused by extreme physical exertion which ruptures the capillaries. This may happen after a severe bout of coughing or sneezing or, in the elderly, may be due to degenerative fragility of the capillaries. Any direct injury may also cause haemorrhage.

The appearance is characteristic with a bright red patch on the conjunctiva which may persist for two to three weeks. The bright colour is maintained as the blood liberated from the broken capillaries obtains oxygen through the thin conjunctival covering.

There is usually no need for any treatment except to reassure the patient that the redness will disappear. Small conjunctival lacerations due to injury will heal, but a very extensive laceration may require suturing with catgut or silk.

CHEMICAL BURNS

Burns of the conjunctiva are very painful and may be associated with burns of the cornea with subsequent scarring which may endanger sight.

The patient will often arrive from an industrial concern in which he is working and where he will have received first aid treatment. Besides being in considerable pain he is likely to be very much afraid of the

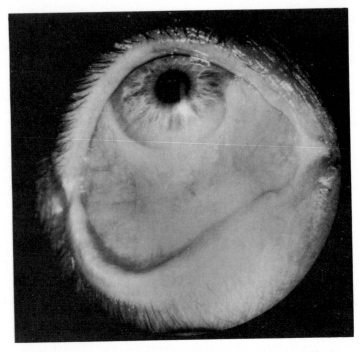

Fig. 40. *Symblepharon from lower lid to eyeball and nasally from eyeball to cornea*

further effect that the burn may have on his eyesight. Besides prompt treatment he will need sympathetic understanding from the nursing staff. Some chemical agents can cause severe damage, the most common being lime which is present in cement and whitewash. A buffer solution of disodium edetate and sodium bicarbonate is the specific antidote for this type of burn.

The burns usually involve the lower bulbar conjunctiva, as the reflex action of closing the lids is preceded by an upturning of the eye. Where possible the chemical responsible for the injury should be identified and the eye thoroughly irrigated with the specific antidote. If necessary reference should be made to the regional poisons centre. If the specific antidote is not known or is not available, the chemical

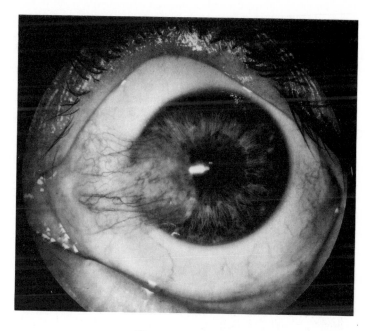

Fig. 41. *Pterygium*

should be diluted and washed out of the conjunctival sac by irrigation with normal saline (see p. 17 for a description of irrigation of the eye).

Burning of the bulbar and palpebral conjunctiva may cause symblepharon (Fig. 40) between the two surfaces, preventing correct closure of the lids and consequently exposing the cornea. Prevention of the formation of symblepharon can be achieved by rodding, when a lubricated glass rod is passed between the two conjunctival surfaces to break down any adhesions that are forming and prevent the formation of further adhesions.

Where there are severe burns it may be necessary to reform the conjunctival sac with grafts of mucous membrane.

It is important to remember that the simple procedure of irrigation is an extremely painful process particularly when treating a lime burn. After irrigation, fluorescein staining of the cornea is carried out and if there is extensive corneal involvement the patient will be admitted to hospital. Otherwise he will attend daily for treatment either at the hospital or at the occupational health centre at his work. The daily treatment of chemical burns is carried out by passing a glass rod round the fornices until healing is complete (see p. 24 for a full description of this procedure).

CONCRETIONS

Inflammatory or degenerative products accumulate as concretions in the crypts of the palpebral conjunctiva. They usually remain as harmless white spots, but may cause irritation if they project beyond the surface, when they can be removed easily with a sharp instrument such as a Saunders' needle.

PINGUECULA

Pinguecula are yellow coloured, slightly raised masses in the conjunctiva on either one or both sides of the cornea which occur after middle age and are left untreated.

PTERYGIUM

A thickening of the bulbar conjunctiva is called pterygium (Fig. 41); it is usually more marked on the nasal side. It is triangular in shape and very vascular; the apex invades the cornea. This condition follows persistent exposure to dust and wind and is common in people who have lived in the Middle East or in Australia. If the cornea has been invaded the tissue is shaved from the cornea and if necessary an overlay corneal graft is carried out.

10

The Lacrimal Apparatus

The lacrimal apparatus is concerned with the production of tears and their drainage through the lacrimal passages to the inferior meatus of the nose. The system consists of the lacrimal glands and their ducts, lacrimal canaliculi, lacrimal sac and the nasolacrimal duct (Fig. 42).

The lacrimal gland is usually described as being the shape and size of an almond and is situated in the upper and lateral of part of the orbit. There are between eight and twelve openings, or lacrimal ducts, which drain the tears into the upper and lateral aspect of the conjunctival fornix. There is very little production of tears in the first few weeks of life and in old age tear production also is reduced.

The function of the tears is to bathe and lubricate the eye. They are composed of 98% water, 1.5% sodium chloride (which gives to the tears their salty flavour) and an enzyme, lysozyme, which has an important antibacterial effect. Repeated irrigations of the eye will dilute the enzyme and lessen its effectiveness and thus it is not desirable for individuals to wash out their eyes regularly.

Sjögren's disease is a condition in which the patient complains of dry eyes and mouth and is the result of a general glandular atrophy particularly affecting the lacrimal and salivary glands. Similarly, in patients with severe chronic conjunctival inflammation, for example trachoma, the lacrimal ducts may become obstructed leading to dryness of the eyes.

In order to diagnose the amount of tears being produced Schirmer's
test is carried out. A small strip of filter paper 50 mm long and 4 mm
wide is folded with a 5 mm turn at one end which is inserted inside the

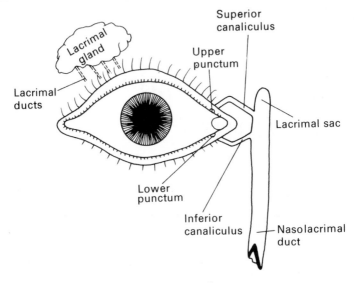

Fig. 42. *The lacrimal apparatus*

lower lid. The patient is asked to keep both eyes closed for five minutes,
when the filter paper is removed. The flow of tears is assessed by the
length of dampened filter paper; anything less than 15 mm is considered
to be below normal. The test is carried out for each eye.

Dry eye is treated by instilling artificial tears. A solution of methylcellulose is a commonly used and effective corneal wetting agent.

From the upper fornix the tears are guided to the medial aspect
of the eye into the puncta, the minute openings of the lacrimal canaliculi in the lid margins. Each canaliculus is about 10 mm long and the
upper and lower canaliculi unite and open into the lacrimal sac.

The lacrimal sac lies on the medial wall of the orbit and is the blind
upper part of the nasolacrimal duct. This duct is about 18 mm long and
3 mm diameter and passes downwards and backwards to empty under
the inferior turbinate bone.

The lacrimal passages are lined by a mucous membrane which is
continuous with the nasal mucosa. Under normal circumstances the

amount of tears formed is sufficient to moisten the eye, and after some evaporation the residual fluid is drained away through the lacrimal passages to the nose.

Undue watering of the eye may be due to:

1. An excessive amount of tears with which the normal system of drainage cannot cope—lacrimation.
2. An obstruction of the lacrimal passages so that the normal amount of tears is not drained away—epiphora.

Lacrimation is usually the result of a reflex stimulation causing the gland to secrete more tears; for example, a corneal foreign body causes excessive watering and is an attempt by the body to rid the eye of the irritant. Emotional stimulation and the peeling of onions are other causes of lacrimation.

Epiphora is a more serious condition as persistent watering of the eye can cause great discomfort, particularly in cold, windy weather, and may also be a source of social embarrassment. The patency of the lacrimal passages may be tested in various ways.

SYRINGING

Normal saline is introduced into the lacrimal sac, using a syringe to which a special cannula is attached (see Figs 9 and 11). Where there is a blockage or partial obstruction of the lacrimal passages the normal saline will not run down into the nose and throat or will only do so if undue pressure is exerted. (For details of this procedure see p. 23.)

DACRYOCYSTOGRAPHY

The lacrimal passages are outlined with radio-opaque liquid, such as Lipiodol, so that their patency can be examined radiographically.

FLUORESCEIN TEST

If function is normal the instillation of fluorescein drops into the conjunctival sac will be followed by detection of the substance in the nasal secretions. This is a quick but not very accurate test.

CONGENITAL OBSTRUCTIONS

Congenital obstructions of the lacrimal ducts may be the result of failure of the ducts to become canalized or of a defective valve mechanism at the lower end of the duct causing an accumulation of lacrimal and conjunctival secretions which can become infected.

A blocked tear duct is usually noticeable a few weeks after birth when one or both eyes will be discharging. When the baby is examined the lacrimal sac may be distended; pressure on the swelling will result in the discharge of mucopurulent material through the punctum—a mucocele.

Treatment

Treatment is by regular expression of the sac. The mother should be taught to swab the eye gently and then exert pressure on the skin at the medial part of the lower lid to express the contents of the sac down the nasolacrimal duct. Antibiotic drops are not effective.

If the condition persists it is necessary to pass a probe into the sac via the canaliculus. The procedure is usually carried out when the child is between six months and one year old and involves admission to the ward for one day, as a general anaesthetic is administered. When the procedure is discussed with the mother it is important to stress that no food or fluid should be given for four hours before operation so that the morning feed is omitted usually and the child brought to the hospital fasting. It is to be hoped that the mother may be allowed to remain at the hospital until the child is ready to go home on recovery from the anaesthetic.

ACQUIRED OBSTRUCTIONS

Acquired obstructions are often the result of inflammation—dacryocystitis. Recurrent dacryocystitis may result in complete obliteration of the sac. This is more often seen in women and after middle age. There is a collection of pus or mucopus in the lacrimal sac causing obstruction and regurgitation of the material. The onset is sudden with a painful swelling over the area of the sac. This may respond to treatment with systemic antibiotics, but sometimes an abscess forms which either may rupture spontaneously or require incision.

If this condition recurs removal of the lacrimal sac, dacryocystectomy, may be advised to prevent further infection, but this operation does not relieve the epiphora. Dacryocystectomy is more suitable for elderly persons who will have a normal reduction of tear production and who may not be fit enough to undergo a prolonged general anaesthetic.

The more effective surgical procedure is dacryocystorrhinostomy in which the lacrimal sac is anastomosed to the nasal mucosa after removal of a portion of the intervening bone. This is a major undertaking but produces good results.

Preoperative Care

The patient undergoing dacryocystorrhinostomy requires general preparation for operation under general anaesthesia. Local preparation varies, but many surgeons like the nose to be packed with ribbon gauze soaked in a solution of 4% cocaine with adrenaline 1:10 000 to bring about constriction of the blood vessels and shrinkage of the nasal mucosa. Bleeding during the operation will obscure the view, particularly when a very small operative site is involved.

Postoperative Care

When the patient has returned to the ward it is important to record the blood pressure at regular intervals until it has reached normal levels as hypotensive drugs are usually used in the theatre in these cases further to promote haemostasis.

A pressure dressing will have been applied over the wound and this must be observed for bleeding. The dressing is removed 24—48 hours after operation and the wound then left uncovered. Since the patient's physical condition is normally satisfactory he may be allowed up. Daily syringing of the passages with normal saline begins on the third day after operation and continues until discharge from hospital unless polyurethane or silicone tubes have been inserted to keep the passages patent. These are left in position for six months. The skin sutures are removed on the fifth postoperative day.

The patient must be told not to blow his nose until healing has taken place and he should be discouraged from wearing spectacles since the weight of the spectacle frames may depress the incision and damage the anastomosis. The patient will need encouragement during this rather trying period. He will be discharged from hospital at the end of a week and given an appointment to attend the clinic after two further weeks.

TRAUMA

Sometimes trauma causes obstruction to the lacrimal passages. Damage to the canaliculi may occur when an animal, most likely a dog, jumps up and tears the face in the region of the lower lid. Surgery may be undertaken to anastomose the torn canaliculi and in such instances fine polythene tubing is inserted to maintain patency; it will be left in position for six months. The tube is threaded through both canaliculi and the ends come out of the nose.

11

Extraocular Muscles

The extraocular muscles of the eyes are concerned with the movements of each eye and in normal vision both are coordinated. There are six muscles: four recti or straight muscles and two oblique (Fig. 43).

RECTI MUSCLES

The *superior rectus* arises near the apex of the orbit, passes forwards and is inserted in the upper surface of the sclera. Its action is to rotate the eye upwards and inwards.

The *inferior rectus* arises near the apex of the orbit, passes forward below the eye and is inserted on the lower surface of the sclera. Its action is to rotate the eye downwards and inwards.

The *medial rectus* arises near the apex of the orbit, passes forward is is inserted in the medial surface of the sclera. Its action is to rotate the eye inwards.

The *lateral rectus* arises near the apex of the orbit and is inserted in the lateral surface of the sclera. Its action is to rotate the eye outwards.

OBLIQUE MUSCLES

The *superior oblique* arises near the apex of the orbit, passes forward along the roof of the orbit where it hooks round the trochlea (or pulley) then passes backwards and outwards and is inserted into the outer

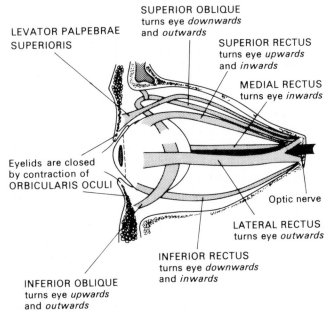

Fig. 43. *The muscles of the eye. The eye is moved by small muscles which link the sclera to the bony orbit. Acting together, the extrinsic muscles can bring about rotatory movement. Both eyes normally move together so that images fall on corresponding points of both retinae*

surface of the sclera behind the equator (midportion of the eye). The effect of this pulley action is to cause the muscle to rotate the eye downwards and inwards.

The *inferior oblique* arises at the lower border of the orbit, passes outwards and is inserted into the lower aspect of the sclera behind the equator. Its action is to rotate the eye upwards and outwards.

The muscles are ensheathed by fascia which covers the the sclera as Tenon's capsule (see p. 11). In every movement of the eyeball several muscles act together and the eyes are maintained in a parallel position by a complicated conditioned reflex which is acquired in early childhood. Man is capable of binocular vision, that is he sees one view with both eyes, the two images being fused together for full stereoscopic vision.

The cranial nerves supply the extraocular muscles. The third cranial or oculomotor nerve supplies the superior, medial and inferior recti and the inferior oblique muscles. The fourth cranial or trochlear nerve supplies the superior oblique muscles. The sixth cranial or abducent nerve supplies the lateral rectus muscle.

STRABISMUS

A strabismus (or squint) is the most common condition affecting the extraocular muscles and is a deviation of the eyes so that their axes are no longer parallel. Most commonly the eyes deviate horizontally either to converge or diverge. A squint may be accompanied by diplopia (double vision).

A *paralytic squint* tends to occur more often in adults and is due to muscle or nerve damage which may be the result of brain injury, intracranial haemorrhage or cerebral tumour. It is essential, therefore, to identify and where possible treat the underlying cause and all persons presenting with such a squint must be investigated carefully. The patient often states that diplopia (double vision) is the most troublesome and distressing symptom. When the patient looks in the direction of the affected muscle the diplopia may be particularly troublesome. It may also lead to giddiness and nausea. The patient often attempts to lessen this symptom by shutting or covering the affected eye. Spectacles may be prescribed to help reduce the diplopia and cosmetic correction of the squint may be carried out later.

In young children, and particularly in infants under the age of six months, the eyes do not work together and so a child may appear to squint; this is known as *concomitant squint*. As full binocular vision is achieved the squint is no longer seen, but it is not too early to examine the eyes for a true squint after the infant reaches six months.

If vision is poor in one eye binocular vision is not possible and one eye will tend to deviate. If this deviation is allowed to persist the vision in the squinting eye will be impaired, producing a 'lazy' or amblyopic eye. The longer the squinting is allowed to continue the more difficult will be successful corrective treatment.

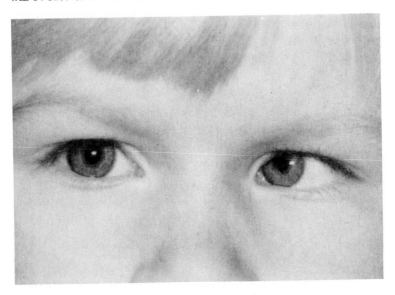

Fig. 44. *A convergent squint*

Epicanthus (a vertical fold of skin at the inner canthus of the eye) up to the age of about four years may give the appearance of a squint although the eyes are normal (Fig. 45).

Treatment

Treatment should be commenced as early as possible. Refraction to estimate the extent of any refractive error will be carried out by the ophthalmologist and suitable spectacles prescribed where necessary. Education or re-education for binocular vision will be necessary and may include the occlusion of the normal eye to strengthen the 'lazy' eye. In addition surgical procedures may be necessary.

The child is referred to the orthoptist who has an important role to play in the treatment of squints. An orthoptist is a recognized medical auxiliary who has been trained and is registered to function as an ocular physiotherapist. The orthoptist will teach the child special exercises which contribute to the development of biocular vision. The

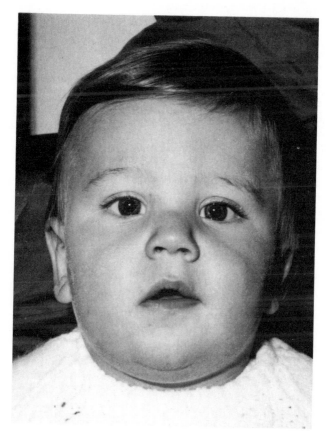

Fig. 45. *An epicanthic fold simulating squint*

orthoptic exercises may be part of the preoperative and postoperative treatment of a patient requiring surgery for the correction of a strabismus.

If a squint persists after correction of the visual defect by spectacles an operation may be needed to realign the squinting eye. Surgical correction of a strabismus is usually carried out when the child is between four and five years of age since by then he will be able to cooperate in the orthoptic exercises.

Preoperative Care

The nursing care of the child admitted to hospital for this operation is that of a child admitted for any surgical procedure under anaesthetic. At this age it is perhaps not so necessary to admit the mother with the child where this is possible and practicable, but free visiting should be allowed. It is always desirable that a child be nursed in a children's hospital or ward rather than in an adult ward.

There is a little special preparation of the eye, apart from the instillation of antibiotic drops preoperatively. If the eyelashes are to be cut, this is done after the child has been anaesthetized as the procedure is otherwise very frightening.

The Operation

There are a number of surgical techniques, but the two most common are:

1. *Recession.* This involves the reinsertion of the muscle farther back on the globe.
2. *Resection.* Here a shortening of the muscle is carried out. The sutures used are of catgut which, since they will become absorbed, do not have to be removed.

Postoperative Care

After operation the child is returned to the ward where he receives the normal close observation and care given after any anaesthetic. Postoperative sedation is seldom necessary following correction of strabismus.

It is more usual to leave the operated eye uncovered as a pad over the eye causes irritation and the child will rub his eye. He may be discharged from hospital one to two days after operation, the mother being given a simple explanation of how to instil the antibiotic drops that will have been ordered.

An appointment will usually be given for the child to attend the clinic one week after discharge from hospital. In the meantime, since there is a tendency for eyes to converge when looking at close objects, the child should be discouraged from reading or watching television until he has been examined again. The eye will be red and this will cause the mother to be concerned; she should be reassured that the redness will subside in two or three weeks, but it should be emphasized that if she is more worried she should contact the hospital before the date of the next appointment.

12

The Protective Structures

THE BONY ORBIT

The orbit (Fig. 46) accommodates the eye and affords its greatest protection, particularly the posterior segment.

Each orbit is roughly cone-shaped with the apex, which is directed backwards and inwards, pierced by a large opening, the optic foramen, through which pass the optic nerve and the ophthalmic artery. The base is directed outwards and forwards and forms a strong bony edge which helps to protect the eyeball.

Each orbit is composed of a roof, floor and medial and lateral walls formed by seven bones with some of the bones shared. These seven are the malar, superior maxillary, palatine, lacrimal, ethmoid, sphenoid and frontal; the last three are shared by both orbits (Fig. 46).

Within the orbit lie the eyeball and optic nerve, the extrinsic ocular muscles, the lacrimal gland, blood vessels and nerves. The spaces between these structures are filled with fat and fascia. A layer of fascia known as Tenon's capsule surrounds the globe of the eye from the cornea to the posterior segment and separates the eye from the orbital fat. The extraocular muscles pierce this capsule.

The posterior portion of the orbit has three openings which lead to the cranial cavity for the transmission of blood vessels and nerves. In addition to this communication between the orbit and the cavity within the skull there are communications through the opening at the apex with the nasal fossae and the accessory nasal sinuses including the air cells of the ethmoidal, sphenoidal, frontal and maxillary bones.

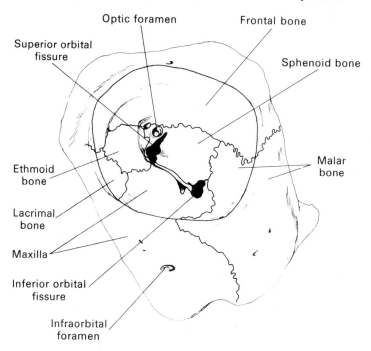

Fig. 46. *Bones forming the left orbit*

The following points are important to remember when considering the anatomy of the orbit.

The superior maxillary bone forms the main part of the floor of the orbit with only 0.5–1 mm of bone between the maxillary sinus and the orbit. Tumours of the antrum may invade the orbit and cause proptosis of the eye.

The medial wall is roughly oblong in shape and is very thin. It is formed by the superior maxillary, lacrimal and ethmoid bones. Because of the thinness of the wall, infection from the ethmoidal air cells may invade the orbit and ethmoiditis is the most common cause of orbital cellulitis.

The lateral wall is triangular in shape and is formed anteriorly by the malar bone and posteriorly by the greater wing of the sphenoid. This lateral wall is the thickest, particularly at the orbital margin where the wall is most exposed to injury.

ORBITAL CELLULITIS

Orbital cellulitis is a serious condition that is usually unilateral and may follow a purulent infection of the orbital cellular tissue. The causes may be infection following a penetrating wound of the orbit, with an airgun pellet for instance, or by spread of infection from a neighbouring structure such as the nasal sinus. It has already been mentioned that ethmoiditis is the most common cause of orbital cellulitis.

Symptoms

The patient appears to be acutely ill with pyrexia which may be accompanied by rigors. There is marked exophthalmos, injection and oedema of the lids and severe pain which is worse when the eye is moved. Abscess formation may either point to the skin of the eyelids or it may discharge through the conjunctival fornix. There is a risk of the infection involving the entire contents of the eyeball—panophthalmitis.

Treatment

The patient is admitted to hospital and is usually nursed in a side ward away from the surgical patients to avoid the risk of cross-infection. Precautions to prevent carrying infection will be taken by nurses who are also involved with other patients.

After the usual details have been taken from the patient or an accompanying relative, the doctor will carry out a careful general and ophthalmic examination. A local and systemic course of a broad-spectrum antibiotic will be started immediately after a swab of any infected material has been taken for culture and sensitivity tests.

The patient should be nursed in bed in whatever position he finds to be most comfortable. He must be encouraged to drink plenty of fluids and, although a light diet may be given, during the first few days of acute illness the patient may have no appetite. Analgesics will be necessary and night sedation is also likely to be required. Application of local heat may help to relieve the discomfort to some extent; if hot spoon bathing is employed there must be supervision by the nurse as otherwise an ill patient may be in danger of scalding himself (see p. 20 for a description of the technique of hot spoon bathing).

While the pyrexia is present and for as long after as required by the doctor the patient's temperature with his pulse and respiration rates should be recorded four-hourly. A note should be made of any rigors, their severity and duration. When the patient's temperature has returned to normal and the infection is subsiding he may be allowed to get up.

Any local cause of the cellulitis is identified and treated. Abscess formation may require incision and drainage, although this is rarely necessary today with intensive antibiotic treatment.

CAVERNOUS SINUS THROMBOSIS

Cavernous sinus thrombosis can occur as a rare and serious complication of orbital cellulitis or the infection may enter the sinus directly from the blood stream or from some other focus of infection. The cavernous sinus is a venous channel lying on either side of the sphenoid bone into which drain the veins of the brain and those of the orbit. Infection can thus be spread into the cranial cavity.

A cavernous sinus thrombosis is one of the few conditions met with in ophthalmic nursing when the patient is critically ill and, if necessary, the relatives must be made aware of the gravity of the illness.

Symptoms

There are proptosis, absence of accommodation and insensivity of the cornea resulting from the involvement of the cranial nerves supplying the eye.

Treatment

The outcome can prove fatal unless intensive treatment is undertaken. An ophthalmologist and physician may together decide upon the line of treatment. Antibiotics are required to treat the infection and anti-coagulants to prevent the formation of septic emboli. The patient needs complete nursing care in bed, including the recording of temperature, pulse and respiration as often as ordered (usually four-hourly); a specimen of urine is tested daily to detect the presence of any blood which may result from the use of anticoagulant drugs (any other bleeding, such as epistaxis, must be reported). Pressure areas should be treated four-hourly and attention paid to oral toilet. A daily bed bath is given. Nursing care aims at making the patient as comfortable as is possible, both physically and mentally.

EXOPHTHALMOS AND PROPTOSIS

Any space-occupying lesion of the bony orbit will push the eyeball forward and will present as an exophthalmos; when there is also pro-tusion of the eyelids the condition is referred to as proptosis. The patient will complain of diplopia if there is a lesion caused by a tumour at the side of the orbit.

Exophthalmos is most commonly met with as a result of endocrine disease. Thyrotoxic exophthalmos is seen in patients with overactivity of the thyroid gland as a result of the action of thyroxine on the orbital muscles.

The signs include delay in closure of the eyelids (lid lag) and, in severe cases, the cornea may be exposed during sleep. In treating such cases paroleine eye drops are instilled at night to protect the cornea.

In some patients treatment of the general disease does not improve the eye symptoms. This is usually the case when there is severe ex-ophthalmos with oedema of the conjunctiva and lids; oedema and fibrosis of the ocular muscles are present. In these patients it may be necessary for a tarsorrhaphy to be performed in order to protect the cornea.

FRACTURES OF THE ORBIT

Fractures may involve damage to the bone and soft tissue and are usually caused by injury with a blunt object.

There is obvious irregularity of outline of the orbit with displacement of the eye. This is most noticeable in fractures of the orbital floor when the inferior rectus muscle can be involved. There is marked tenderness and emphysema of the subcutaneous tissue.

Treatment

Treatment depends upon the severity and degree of the injury. Orbital cellulitis may be a complicating factor.

A radiographic examination is necessary to determine the extent of the damage. The wounds are cleaned and sutured and antitetanus toxoid given. If foreign bodies, for example pellets, are in the orbit it may be safer to leave them rather than run the risk of causing further damage by removing them.

When the floor of the orbit has been fractured any surgical reconstruction is delayed until haematoma formation and emphysema have subsided. The orbit may then be lined with a toughened silicone sheeting in the area of the fracture. Patients who have extensive fractures of the orbit and face are usually transferred to the regional faciomaxillary centre.

TUMOURS

Tumours are not common but they may arise from the walls or from the contents of the orbit. Deep X-ray therapy and irradiation techniques are the usual method of treatment and such patients are referred to a radiotherapy centre. Surgical intervention is sometimes necessary. (See also Burkitt's lymphoma, p. 162.)

EYELIDS AND EYELASHES

The eyelids and eyelashes play a very important part in the protective mechanism of the eye.

The eyelids are formed by two movable folds of skin with an anterior, or skin surface and a posterior, or conjunctival surface which are connected by the lid margins. Each lid also has an orbital and palpebral

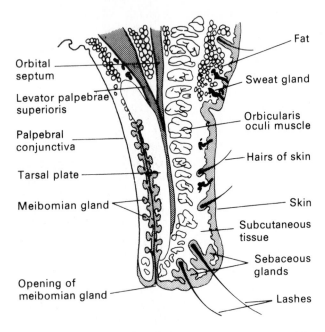

Orbital septum

Levator palpebrae superioris

Palpebral conjunctiva

Tarsal plate

Meibomian gland

Opening of meibomian gland

Fat

Sweat gland

Orbicularis oculi muscle

Hairs of skin

Skin

Subcutaneous tissue

Sebaceous glands

Lashes

Fig. 47. *Longitudinal section through the upper eyelid*

portion. In the upper lid the orbital portion extends from the eyebrow to cover the upper part of the orbit and the palpebral portion covers the upper part of the eyeball. In the lower lid the orbital portion extends from the cheek to cover the lower part of the eyeball.

At the skin surface of the lid margin is an anterior lip in which the eyelashes are inserted. A grey line appears behind the lashes which is important in surgery as it divides the anterior and posterior portions of the lid. The conjunctival surface is separated from the lid margin by the posterior lip and close to this posterior lip are situated the meibomian glands. These are sebaceous glands filled with a fatty secretion which lubricates the lid margin and prevents overspill of the normal flow of tears from the conjunctival sac. They also form a surface layer of precorneal fluid which prevents undue evaporation of the tears from the surface of the cornea. The structure of the upper lid is shown in Fig. 47.

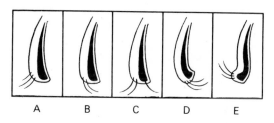

Fig. 48. *Section of the upper eyelid showing normal and abnormal positions of the tarsus and lashes. A, Normal eyelid. B, Trichiasis. C, Distichiasis. D, Entropion, E, Ectropion*

The upper and lower lids meet at an angle at the medial and lateral canthus. At the medial aspect of the lid margins are small perforated raised areas, the puncta, which form the entrance to the lacrimal ducts. At the medial canthus is the rounded vascular structure, the caruncle.

The hair follicles carrying the eyelashes are situated within the loose connective tissue and muscular layer. The glands of Zeis are sebaceous glands which are associated with the hair follicles and the glands of Moll sweat glands whose ducts enter into or near the hair follicle. There is some degree of rigidity of the lids due to the dense fibrous tissue of which the tarsal plate is composed.

BELL'S PHENOMENON

Bell's phenomenon is the updrawing movement of the eye before the lids are closed fully. It may be observed in ectropion and some other lid deformities where loss of tissue has taken place.

DISTICHIASIS

Distichiasis (Fig. 48C) is a rare condition in which the meibomian glands fail to develop and are replaced by a row of lashes which turn in and irritate the cornea. These lashes can be removed by electrolysis, destroying the follicles.

EPICANTHUS

The epicanthus is a broad fold of skin from the base of the nose to the eyebrows which tends to obscure the medial canthus and increases the breadth of the nose. The epicanthus is normally seen in babies but, in the majority of children, it disappears as the face develops. However, persistence of the fold is characteristic of Mongoloid races and patients suffering from Down's syndrome.

Foreign bodies frequently become lodged on the conjunctival surface of the upper lid and are referred to as subtarsal foreign bodies. They constitute one of the most common complaints met with in casualty departments. Removal of the foreign body is made easier by eversion of the upper lid (see Fig. 5). Any particle of, for example, grit adherent to the subtarsal surface of the lid may cause damage to the cornea, as each time the patient blinks the grit scratches the corneal surface.

Practise is needed to acquire facility in everting the upper lid (see p. 16). Pressure on the eyeball must be avoided for it causes the patient discomfort and he will react by squeezing the lids shut.

Eversion of the lower lid is carried out by simply drawing the lower lid down and asking the patient to look up.

MUSCLES OF THE EYELIDS

There are two muscles concerned in the opening and closing of the lids:

1. The *levator palpabrae*, which is a voluntary muscle supplied by the third cranial nerve, the action of which is to raise the upper lid.
2. The *orbicularis oculi*, supplied by the seventh cranial nerve (the facial nerve), the action of which is to close the lids. The palpebral portion is used for gentle closure and the orbital portion for forcible closure of the lids.

PTOSIS

A congenital abnormality in which drooping of one or both upper lids occurs in ptosis; it is the result of a developmental defect of the levator muscle. In severe unilateral cases there may be some amblyopia ('lazy eye') as the eye is not used. When there is bilateral ptosis the child will tip his head back in order to look from under the drooping lids. Surgery for this deformity is usually resection of the levator palpabrae superioris. The incision is either through the skin (Everbusch's operation) or through the conjunctiva (Blaskovic's operation). Head posture often has to be corrected after surgery as the child will have acquired the habit of tilting the head back.

Acquired ptosis may be seen in myasthenia gravis or may be a senile myasthenia when the lax tissues of old age tend to sag.

BLEPHARITIS

Blepharitis, a chronic inflammatory condition of the lid margins, can be described as squamous or ulcerative.

Squamous or non-ulcerative blepharitis is characterized by redness and swelling of the lid margins with a fine powdery deposit or scales on the lashes and a tendency for them to fall out. It is frequently associated with a seborrhoeic dermatitis and is often seen in children and adolescents; rubbing of the eyelids to relieve the irritation aggravates the condition, as may exposure to a smoky atmosphere and cosmetics. Advice should be given where appropriate on the use of make-up.

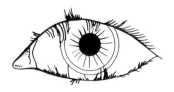

Fig. 49. *Trichiasis of the upper eyelid and entropion of the lower*

Ulcerative blepharitis develops as the result of a secondary staphylococcal infection and if it is allowed to persist will cause a permanent distortion of the eyelash follicles and subsequent inturning lashes (trichiasis) (Fig. 49) which may result in corneal ulceration. The condition may arise in part from poor hygiene and malnutrition and it is important that where this is so teaching in proper hygiene and attention to diet should be given.

Local treatment consists of keeping the lid margins free of crusting and scales by swabbing and the use of antibiotics. (A description of swabbing will be found on p.13.) A topical steroid may be used to treat the inflammation but must be used only in conjunction with the appropriate antibacterial treatment.

STYE (EXTERNAL HORDEOLUM)

A stye (external hordeolum) (Fig. 50) is an infection of the eyelash follicle or the sebaceous glands associated with it. The infected area becomes red, swollen and painful and eventually a yellow 'head' develops which points along the line of the lash and ruptures with the release of purulent discharge. Styes often recur and may be associated with blepharitis. The application of moist heat in the form of hot spoon bathing may serve to hasten the formation of the head of the stye followed by the discharge of pus.

MEIBOMIAN CYST

A meibomian cyst (Fig. 51) presents as a small, firm swelling within a meibomian gland and is caused by blockage of the gland with sebaceous material. The enlargement is halted after a few days as the accumulated material blocks the secreting cells of the gland. The cyst becomes a round, painless projection on the conjunctival surface of the lid. When the lid is everted a reddened area is seen which, if large, may cause corneal irritation. Occasionally there is secondary infection with accompanying pain and oedema.

Treatment

Sometimes a meibomian cyst may subside spontaneously after a few weeks, but usually it is necessary for the cyst to be incised and the contents curretted. If there is secondary infection hot spoon bathing and the application of an antibiotic ointment will be ordered.

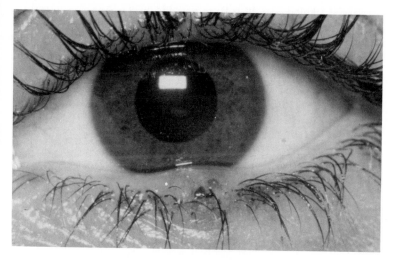

Fig. 50. *A stye (external hordeolum)*

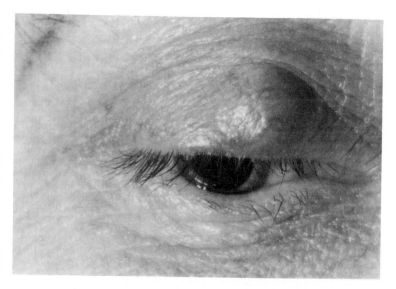

Fig. 51. *A meibomian cyst (internal hordeolum)*

Surgical treatment is usually carried out under local anaesthesia at a minor operations session in the out-patient department. The patient should be told that this is a minor operation of short duration and that, as he will wear a pad and bandage over the eye for a few hours afterwards, he will be unable to drive a car home.

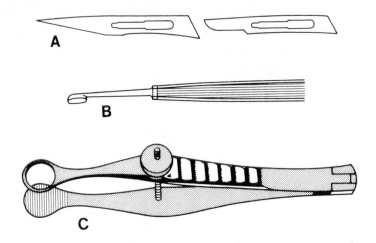

Fig. 52. *Equipment for the removal of a meibomian cyst.*
A, Small scalpel blades. B, A meibomian cyst scoop.
C, A meibomian cyst clamp

On arrival for the procedure the patient will be made comfortable, preferably lying down on a couch; if he is very nervous it is helpful if a nurse can stand beside him to reassure him. During the procedure the lid is everted with a meibomian clamp; a vertical incision is made away from the lid margin and the contents are curretted out. When the clamp is released some bleeding will take place so that a firm pad and bandage is applied to the closed eye and the patient kept under observation for about half an hour before going home. The pad and badage should then be left in position for about four hours after which it can be removed and the eye bathed gently with warm saline. The patient or an accompanying relative or friend will have been instructed how to do this. The eye will most likely appear bruised for several days and the patient may wish to wear dark glasses until the bruising has subsided.

ALLERGIC DERMATITIS

The lids can be affected by external agents which produce an allergic response in a sensitized subject; there may be a moist eczema and oedematous swelling of the skin with irritation. The cause of the sensitivity may be any one of a host of substances, including drugs such as atropine or penicillin, cosmetics such as mascara or metals such as the nickel used in spectacle frames.

It is sometimes possible to identify the cause of the sensitivity by patch testing; the patient can then be warned to avoid further contact. Treatment consists of the removal of the offending substance and the use of topical steroids.

ABNORMAL POSITIONS OF THE LID MARGINS

Ectropion

In ectropion (Fig. 48E) the lower lid margin is everted so that it is no longer in contact with the surface of the eye; the palpebral conjunctiva is exposed and there is persistent epiphora. The main cause of this abnormality is loss of muscle tone and thus it is common in the elderly, but it may also be seen in patients who have had facial injuries with scar tissues in the region of the lids. The condition is aggravated by a tendency to wipe the lid in a downward direction.

Various forms of muscle shortening operation have been devised to correct the defect. Patients usually attend a minor operations session in the out-patient department.

Entropion

In entropion (Fig. 48D) the lid margin is inverted so that the lashes rub against the eyeball. The condition may be caused by a spasm of the orbicularis oculi caused by irritation of the eye or it may follow scarring of the lid.

A strip of adhesive plaster from the lid margin to the cheek may be sufficient to correct the defect. Cautery to the muscle will cause scarring and prevent spasm, or more complicated plastic surgery may be required.

HERPES ZOSTER OPHTHALMICUS

Herpes zoster ophthalmicus is a very painful condition which is seen usually in middle or old age and which may cause scarring of the cornea (Fig. 53). It is a virus infection affecting the ophthalmic division of the trigeminal nerve and is related to the viruses of chicken pox and herpes simplex.

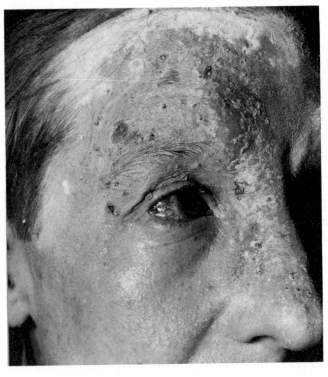

Fig. 53. *Herpes zoster ophthalmicus*

The first symptom is pain along the distribution of the nerve—the scalp, forehead, upper eyelid and tip of the nose if the nasociliary branch of the nerve is affected. This is the external nasal nerve which not only supplies the nose but is the sensory nerve of the eyeball. The skin over the area becomes swollen and there is a vesicular eruption.

The conjunctiva usually becomes red and the cornea may become involved, becoming oedematous and developing vesicles. There may be severe uveitis and secondary glaucoma.

Treatment

In severe cases it is necessary for the patient to be admitted to hospital. He will be nursed in a single room since this is an infective condition, although complete isolation nursing is not usually necessary.

The main problem in caring for these patients is the severe pain they experience. Analgesics such as pethidine and dihydrocodeine (DF118) may be ordered, to be given as required and night sedation is usually necessary. The patients often become depressed by the pain, which may continue for long after the active stage of the disease. The nurse needs to use her skills to support the patient and give him what reassurance she can.

Idoxuridine, which has a specific antiherpetic activity, is used topically. The vesicles on the forehead, lids and elsewhere should be kept dry by the use of calamine lotion and secondary infection avoided by the application of antibiotic ointment. The advice of a dermatologist may be sought in the management of the skin lesions.

Treatment of the eye will also be dependent upon any complication which develop, for example iritis or corneal ulceration. Sometimes it is necessary for a tarsorrhaphy to be performed if corneal involvement has rendered it insensitive.

TUMOURS OF THE EYELID

Tumours commonly occur. A papilloma or benign tumour is usually treated by excision.

A basal cell carcinoma (rodent ulcer) is the most common form of carcinoma of the eyelids. It is usually seen on the lower lid or on the skin around the medial canthus. The tumour may break down and gradually spread but is of a low malignancy and does not metastasize. Many patients do not seek treatment for several years.

Treatment may be surgical excision of the tumour and if necessary plastic repair of the lid. Irradiation is sometimes required. It is customary to follow up these patients at regular intervals for about five years.

EYEBROWS

The eyebrows, which cover the superior orbital ridge, are thickened ridges of skin covered with short hairs. The underlying tissue contains fibres of several muscles including the corrugator which is used in frowning. The occipito frontalis elevates the eyebrows and causes transverse wrinkles of the forehead.

The eyebrows protect the eye from perspiration of the forehead and trap organic and inorganic particles. They may be affected by dandruff falling from the scalp or by an allergic reaction which may be associated with an allergic condition of the eyelids.

13

Ophthalmic Conditions of Tropical Climates

Diseases that are common in one area may be of secondary importance in another, but the relative ease of travel nowadays means that nurses must be better prepared than ever to deal with conditions with which formerly only the specialist needed to be familiar. In this chapter we deal with some of the commoner tropical conditions likely to be encountered, in the United Kingdom as well as overseas, and we have included some generalized diseases in which eye complications may occur.

Conditions of life in tropical countries are often vastly different from those in temperate ones. Glare, heat, humidity, dust, flies and other insects are all commonplace; many bacteria and parasites are widespread, and poverty and malnutrition, poor housing, sanitation and personal hygiene, and inadequate education all conspire to aggravate the adverse conditions. Economic problems in many developing countries make treatment of eye conditions too expensive for the local population. There is also a shortage of trained doctors and nurses in many areas. Such factors, which are often coupled with difficulties in communications and transport, can make the provision of adequate care a very frustrating and sometimes impossible task. Ignorance is prevalent and often patients with eye conditions may be treated in their villages by the introduction into the eye of various substances which can often do much harm. It requires tact and understanding on the part of doctors and nurses to persuade patients and their families to abandon local methods and accept modern medical treatment.

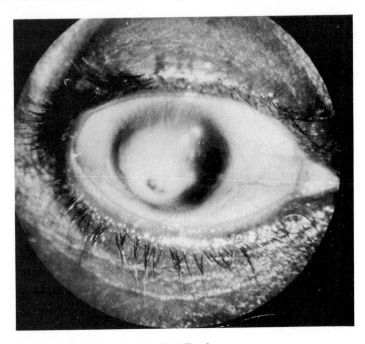

Fig. 54. *Trachoma*

TRACHOMA

It is estimated that there are 400 to 500 million cases of trachoma in the world and of these 125 million are in India alone. Although it may occur in most areas the degree of severity and chronicity seems to be related to socio-economic conditions and to standards of hygiene. Despite the success of numerous control programmes involving extensive health education and treatment of infected persons, trachoma remains the most important single cause of preventable blindness in developing countries.

The name is derived from the Greek word 'trachus' meaning roughness and describes the hard granulations that develop on the inner surface of the eyelids. The causative organism is a virus.

Trachoma is a chronic infective keratoconjunctivitis which first causes thickening of the conjunctiva with the formation of round, translucent follicles. The cornea may also be involved and is invaded by new blood vessels; in the later stages there is corneal scarring. The infective stage may extend for several months or even years but is eventually self-limiting. Although in many patients healing occurs spontaneously the cornea may be further damaged by entropion (abnormal inward displacement of the lid margin) and trichiasis (lashes that turn against the cornea), both of which are the result of scarring of the lids. In fact some permanent scarring of the cornea is inevitable, and loss of vision—total blindness in many cases—will result. At the same time changes continue in the tissues of the lids which may result in symblepharon (adhesion of the lid to the eyeball).

Treatment

Improvements in living standards and personal hygiene are important preventive measures, but it must be remembered that the disease occurs among populations living in extreme poverty when these can not readily be achieved. Controlled health education and mass treatment programmes are necessary to cope with the large numbers of people in affected areas. Local treatment consists of the instillation of chloramphenicol or sulphacetamide drops; broad spectrum antibiotics are also used systemically.

The follicles may be expressed with a special type of roller forceps and cauterization of the lids with silver nitrate or copper sulphate may be necessary. If there is severe corneal scarring, operation to correct deformities of the lids and keratoplasty may be undertaken.

EPIDEMIC KERATOCONJUNCTIVITIS

The causative organism of epidemic keratoconjunctivitis is a virus; it is air-borne and spreads readily in conditions of dust and wind. The disease is endemic in India and the Far East, particularly in summer and autumn, but also occurs in epidemics in the USA and elsewhere.

The condition progresses from a mild conjunctivitis to superficial punctate ulcers of the cornea. Severe and untreated cases may develop disciform keratitis.

Treatment is with normal saline irrigations and mydriatics. Local steroids are not generally used as they delay healing of the cornea and may result in corneal perforation.

FILARIAL INFECTIONS

Filariae are nematodes or roundworms of which the adults of both sexes inhabit lymphatics, connective tissue and mesentery. Large numbers of live embryos or microfilariae are produced which live in the blood stream without further development.

ONCHOCERCIASIS (RIVER BLINDNESS)

Onchocerciasis is a filarial disease which occurs mainly in West Africa and Central America. It is estimated to affect some 20 million people. The male worm is about 4 cm in length and the female can be up to 40 cm.

The adult worms inhabit subcutaneous tissues where they give rise to small fibrous tumours about an 2 cm in diameter in which worms may be found. The embryo microfilaria is about 300 μm long and is found in the skin, especially in the region of the nodules. It is transmitted to humans by the bite of the female 'black flies' which exist in rivers and streams. Hydroelectric schemes create breeding grounds in the spillways of the dams and in downstream sections.

Although it is rare to find the adult worm inside the eyes, invasion with microfilariae is common and in some places almost all the inhabitants of a village may be blind from the disease. The blind adults are led round by young children who in their turn will be led round by other youngsters when they too become infested by the worm. Fluffy punctate patches of keratitis develop until the whole of the centre of the cornea may be involved and vision impaired. Living microfilariae may be seen wriggling in the aqueous with the aid of a slit-lamp. A mass of dead microfilariae in the anterior chamber distorts the pupil which is pear-shaped with the point downwards. Secondary glaucoma and cataract may develop, involvement of the retina and choroid leads to disorganization of these structures and optic atrophy. Local treatment is that of iritis (p. 161), with excision of the nodules. Systemic treatment with diethylcarbamizine will be given if infection is severe; a normal dosage would be 2 mg/kg body weight three times daily for three weeks.

LOA LOA (LOAISIS)

This 'eye worm' is found mainly in West Africa and is transmitted to humans by the bite of a species of horse-fly. The adult worm is about 3 cm long. It works its way through the subcutaneous tissues and may enter the eye, where it is easily seen under the conjunctiva against the white sclera. It travels at the rate of about 1.25 cm a minute.

Cocaine eye drops instilled in the eye partially paralyse the worm, which is then transfixed with needle and thread and gently removed. Systemic treatment with diethylcarbamizine is given.

OPHTHALMIA NEONATORUM

Mucopurulent conjunctivitis is common throughout the world, but is the third commonest eye condition to be found in tropical regions. The disease is notifiable in the United Kingdom as ophthalmia neonatorum if it occurs within 21 days of birth. A fuller discussion of symptoms and treatment is given on p. 121. Nurses working in hot climates where the condition is prevalent must pay particular attention to hygiene. The infection may be transmitted to the babies' eyes by infected swabs or soiled linen after birth, as well as during the passage of the infant down the birth canal.

The causative organisms may be staphylococcus, gonococcus or TRIC virus. The latter causes a condition similar to gonococcal conjunctivitis and appears to be related to trachoma virus.

LYMPHOMA OF THE ORBIT

Burkitt's lymphoma is a highly malignant tumour which, although it is commonest in the jaw and abdomen, may occur in the orbit. It may be the result of infection with Epstein—Barr virus which has been cultured from the tumour tissue. Distribution is between approximately 15° north and south of the equator where temperatures and rainfall are high, and the highest incidence is in Central Africa. The tumour is seen in children between the ages of two and fourteen.

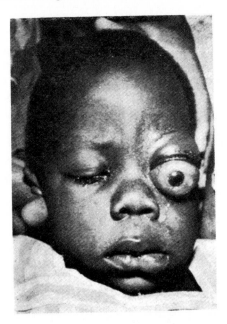

Fig. 55. *Burkitt's lymphoma*

In the eye the tumour is the commonest cause of unilateral exophthalmos in young children in the endemic area. An early sign is oedema of the eyelids followed by marked chemosis; spread within the orbit results in exophthalmos and gross displacement of the eye. The globe is not invaded until the disease is well advanced, and this distinguishes it from retinoblastoma with which it may be confused.

Treatment

The best treatment at present is by cytotoxic drugs such as methotrexate and cyclophosphamide. Radiotherapy has not proved successful.

MALNUTRITION

Malnutrition, which is widespread in many areas, may be a cause of
eye affections and it will adversely affect the patient's resistance to
generalized infection. Neglect, due to apathy, ignorance and lack of
facilities, often aggravates an existing condition so that patients are
often seen only when their illness is in an advanced stage.

In the East and in other parts of the world many thousands are
partially sighted or blind. Although disease such as trachoma, onchocerciasis, trauma or ophthalmia neonatorum account for much of this,
it is becoming increasingly obvious that a great deal of blindness is due
to malnutrition or frank starvation.

Defective day vision may follow malnutrition and is also seen in
lack of vitamin B. Visual acuity may be reduced to 6/60 and if untreated the loss of vision is permanent.

KERATOMALACIA

This condition results from gross deficiency of vitamin A. It is common
in many parts of Asia and Africa and the patient, usually an infant or
young child, will almost certainly be suffering also from malnutrition.

In the early stages the conjunctiva becomes dry and opaque, and
small foam-like white spots may form near the limbus. There is night
blindness. As the condition worsens the cornea becomes involved;
it too becomes dry, insensitive and eventually opaque. Perforation may
occur without any signs of inflammation and this can be followed
rapidly by prolapse of the iris, loss of vitreous and destruction of the
eye. The tissues of the eye become soft and may eventually dissolve and
leak away through the disintegrating cornea.

Both keratomalacia and its early less severe manifestation, xerophthalmia, must be treated urgently with huge doses of vitamin A.

Blindness can develop rapidly—in a matter of days only—and many children die. The incidence in malnourished children is high, possibly as much as 70% or more. All children who appear to be undernourished should be examined for evidence of vitamin A deficiency and eye conditions and treatment should be both immediate and energetic.

SMALLPOX

With active vaccination programmes over many years and the follow-up of any possible contacts smallpox has been eradicated. Some patients may still be seen, who as a result of smallpox with pustules which involved the cornea, suffered severe corneal perforation leading to endophthalmitis and phthisis bulbi.

LEPROSY

Leprosy can be seen in almost all parts of the world although it is particularly prevalent in the tropics. Some 12 to 15 million people are probably infected, with tropical Africa and parts of India having the highest incidence.

Eye involvement is very variable and is influenced by differences in the severity and type of the disease. All structures of the eye can become involved and there may be some difficulty in recognizing the early signs. All patients at risk and those with a confirmed diagnosis of leprosy should have periodic eye examinations by an expert.

The most serious ophthalmic complication is iritis, which may lead to blindness if left untreated. Other structures of the eye may also be affected. All conditions should receive the appropriate local treatment (see pp. 100–109), the patient meanwhile will receive systemic treatment for leprosy. The sulphones used in the systemic treatment of leprosy may cause an allergic reaction in the eye.

OTHER TROPICAL INFECTIONS

Many of the tropical fevers are accompanied by dehydration, which can often be severe. Treatment of any conjunctivitis that may develop with the fever should be started as soon as possible, to prevent the congestion from developing into a conjunctival harmorrhage. In malaria in particular the patient may become partially comatose and in cholera coma the cornea is at particular risk as the patient's eyelids normally remain partially open and unblinking. The cornea should be kept moist and a protective shield can be applied over the eye to keep out dust, glare and further infection. Fevers accompanied by jaundice, for example yellow fever, may provoke retinal haemorrhage, which can be severe.

In summary therefore, the ophthalmic nurse should be especially vigilant when caring for a patient with one of the generalized tropical infections. Complications are not necessarily very different from those encountered elsewhere but they may well be more serious or be seen at more advanced stages. It is perhaps worth restating that many patients in tropical areas will be suffering from malnutrition and that this, together with the dust, flies and poor hygiene that is so often the norm, will leave the eyes more vulnerable and will aggravate any infection that has developed. Indeed, much of the ophthalmic morbidity encountered in the tropics is a direct result of the poverty, ignorance and lack of medical facilities that are so prevalent in many of these areas.

14

Enucleation

Enucleation of an eye involves the removal of the eyeball and is undertaken for the following reasons:

1. A blind, painful eye.
2. An eye which constitutes a danger to the patient's health, for example when there is a possibility of a malignant tumour metastasizing.
3. An eye which has been injured so extensively that repair is impossible, or where there is a risk of the damaged eye causing sympathetic ophthalmia in its undamaged fellow.

The nurse must understand that the removal of an eye is always a severe shock to a patient and she must be prepared to give him especially sympathetic understanding and reassurance. She may expect the patient to ask many questions which she must answer where she can, not hesitating to refer him to the ward sister or the doctor if the questions are beyond her competence.

Patients who have a blind eye which is useless and causing them pain may themselves express the desire to have the eye removed and this will influence the ophthalmic surgeon in deciding whether or not to operate. On the other hand, a patient who has a malignant tumour may have no distressing symptoms in the early stages and a very careful explanation of the need for the operation will have been given by the doctor; the patient may subsequently wish to discuss this with the nurse. Sometimes such a patient may feel unable to accept advice that his eye must be removed and will ask for a second medical opinion and his wish must be understood and respected.

For patients who have developed sympathetic ophthalmia the only hope of recovery of the affected eye is to remove the 'exciting' eye which is often considered by the patient to be his 'good' eye. Here again very careful explanation is necessary.

When enucleation is necessary in a child the nurse must understand the great distress this will cause his parents and be ready to give them as much support as possible; after the doctor has explained the need for such an operation, the nurse should do what she can to help the parents in their distress and anxiety. It is important to remember that a child who is old enough to understand should also be told that his eye is to be removed.

PREOPERATIVE CARE

The psychological care of the patient is very important. When the need for the removal of the eye has been accepted the patient will often ask questions about artificial eyes. He may be very concerned as to whether he will be competent in handling and removing the artificial eye and should be given reassurance that with practise this should not constitute a problem.

Physical preparation for the operation is as for any patient who is to undergo general anaesthesia. The eyelashes are left uncut. It is very important to ensure that there is no confusion over which eye is to be removed. To eliminate the possibility of any error the doctor will mark the forehead over the eye for removal.

POSTOPERATIVE CARE

At the end of the operation a firm pressure dressing is applied to the socket to prevent the formation of a haematoma. The patient is returned to the ward and is cared for in the same way as any patient recovering from a general anaesthetic. Once he is fully recovered and his general condition permits the patient may be allowed to be up and about.

To improve the cosmetic appearance a plastic implant, to which the four recti muscles have been sutured, may be inserted into the socket.

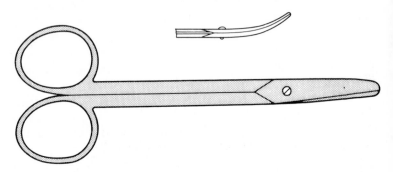

Fig. 56. *Enucleation scissors*

The firm dressing is left in position for 24—48 hours and then removed. There is usually some serous discharge from the socket, which should be bathed gently twice a day with swabs moistened with normal saline or irrigated with normal saline, according to the preference of the surgeon. Where there is no serous discharge the socket is best left uncovered. The patient will feel very conscious of his appearance at this time and he is either given dark glasses to wear or, if he is accustomed to wearing spectacles, the lens over the socket is occluded.

As soon as possible, usually within three of four days, a temporary 'shell' or prosthesis is fitted into the socket. This is done to prevent shrinkage and to accustom the patient to the insertion and removal of the shell before he goes home. When the socket has settled after a few weeks, the shell is replaced by an artificial eye which is also shell-shaped and is specially prepared for that individual patient. Various lenses are shown in Fig. 57.

Discharge from hospital is usually one week after operation and the patient is given appointments to visit the artificial eye fitter and the surgeon.

FITTING A TEMPORARY SHELL OR ARTIFICIAL EYE

On the first occasion of the fitting of a shell or artifical eye the patient will be very tense as he is usually afraid that the procedure will be painful. The nurse should be able to reassure him that although he will feel the presence of something in the eye socket there will be no pain. In some cases surgeons carrying out an enucleation insert an

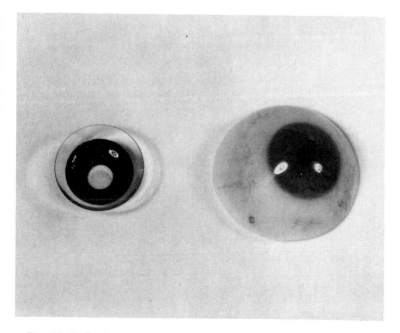

Fig. 57. Left, *A cosmetic soft lens with painted iris and clear pupil.*
Right, *A scleral (haptic) cosmetic lens with a clear pupil*

implant in the socket to which the four recti muscles are attached, covering it with conjunctiva. This will give a better cosmetic effect as the artificial eye, when fitted, will move.

The patient should be allowed to handle the shell or artificial eye to become familiar with its shape. He will notice that the shell has a notch on the nasal side to accommodate the trochlea and this is a useful guide to its correct positioning.

The patient should be seated for the insertion of the shell which is moistened so that it will slip into the socket more easily. The upper lid is raised and the upper edge of the shell slipped under; it is then held in place with the thumb of the left hand whilst the lower lid is drawn down and the lower edge of the shell slipped into the lower fornix.

The seated patient is asked to look up and either a glass rod or the little finger is eased under the lower edge of the shell whilst the lower lid margin is drawn down. Gentle pressure is exerted on the upper lid and the shell will slip out.

Training a patient to undertake these tasks for himself needs care, patience and understanding. At first the patient will feel very nervous and to some people the whole process may be repellent. Practise is best undertaken in the bathroom in front of a mirror. A towel placed in the basin will protect the shell from damage if it slips through the patient's fingers.

By the time he is ready for discharge from hospital the patient should be able to insert and remove the shell with confidence. He should be advised to remove the shell once a day and to clean the socket gently.

EVISCERATION

Evisceration is a method of removing an infected eye. The cornea and contents of the eyeball are removed, but the sclera is left in place with the muscles attached. This operation avoids cutting the optic nerve and thus the risk of infection spreading into the cranial cavity. The present day use of antibiotic drugs has reduced the need for evisceration.

EXENTERATION

Exenteration is a very extensive operation undertaken for some malignant tumours. The lids and entire contents of the orbit are removed. A prosthesis representing eyelids and an eye can be fitted on to a spectacle frame. The cavity is covered with a skin graft.

15

Blindness

A person may be registered as blind if he is unable to perform any work for which eyesight is essential. In the United Kingdom some 116 000 people are registered as blind but of these only a small proportion, about 10%, are totally blind, i.e. not able to differentiate between dark and light. There is no statutory definition of partial sight. In children blindness means that a child's sight is not good enough for learning by sighted methods. In talking about blindness it is often easier to use the term visually handicapped, as this is a better description of the total situation.

Blindness in the United Kingdom is caused mainly by three diseases; cataract, glaucoma and senile degeneration of the macula. There are other conditions that are less common causes of blindness such as optic neuritis, intracranial lesions and accidental trauma.

The Certificate of Registration of blindness is completed by a consultant ophthalmologist who will have examined the person to ascertain the degree of sight and the prognosis. The completed form is sent to the Director of Social Services for the area in which the blind person lives. If the conditions of blindness are fulfilled then the person is certified as blind and his name is added to the register.

BLIND CHILDREN

Every year a number of children suffer from deterioration of sight through illness or accident or as the progression of a sight defect. Children who are born blind usually remain at home to be cared for by their parents with the support of the staff of the social services department or the local education authority. The principal responsibility for the development of the blind child will fall upon the mother since she will be with him for the greater part of the time. Anyone who has the responsibility of caring for a young blind child will want to feel that all possible support and help is made available to him and to his family so that they too may learn to accept and overcome his handicap and that he may become a happy and acceptable member of the community.

Blind children need extra care so that they develop normally. The blind child, for instance, learns to speak later than the sighted child since he is unable to associate words with the viewed objects surrounding him. It is therefore important that he is helped to develop other senses, touch, hearing and smell, to compensate for the lack of sight. The mother of a blind infant and toddler should handle him more than she would a sighted child to give him a sense of security and of growing in a setting of love and care. At the same time she must avoid the pitfall of overprotection and allow him to become as independent as possible.

The statutory period of education for all blind children is from five to 16 years, although many remain in full-time education for longer than this. To bring help to the parents of young blind children and to ensure they have support when they need it most, the education advisory service of the Royal National Institute for the Blind may be the first service to which parents turn. The Institute provides practical help and support to parents. When a blind child reaches the age of three he may benefit from wider experiences or more specialized training such as may be provided in the Sunshine Homes Nursery Schools. Children may be admitted at three years old unless there is a special reason for them being admitted earlier. They can remain there until they are ready to move on to their next school, usually at about the age of six. Time spent in such a Sunshine Home enables an assessment of the child's needs to take place so that recommendation can be made about the child's future placement in a school. It also acts as a bridge between home and the world of school.

Schools for the blind in the United Kingdom form part of the total national educational provision for children. Several of the schools for the blind are maintained by voluntary charitable institutions. It is not compulsory for a blind child to attend a school for the blind if the parents wish him to attend a school for sighted children and if the local education authority is able to arrange for such provision as is needed to support the blind child.

At about 11 years old children are assessed for their suitability for selective secondary education and may either go to a school which prepares them to proceed to university, colleges or professional training or attend a school for the blind or a secondary department of the school which they are already attending. This continues until they leave at 16 or later if they are taking any examinations. On leaving they may go into employment or transfer to one of the vocational assessment centres or a course of further education. It is important that school leavers feel they can be accepted as ordinary members of the community. On leaving school the majority of blind young people seek employment and interests in the ordinary world rather than in sheltered employment. Blind adolescents are often not aware of the wide range of occupations available to them. They may also realize the social restrictions of visual handicap. Residential centres are available to provide the necessary vocational guidance, social adjustment and continuing education for such school leavers.

Facilities are also available for special training to be given at a skills centre or at a special college, e.g. physiotherapy training at the RNIB School in London.

Some blind people continue a course of further or higher education at a technical college, polytechnic or university.

BLIND ADULTS

The adult who has been blind from childhood will have learned to live with his disability and will have received education especially geared to his needs. The newly blinded adult, on the other hand, is in need of special care and support, particularly when the onset of blindness is sudden. Such persons have to orientate themselves to a new way of life and may undergo much suffering, physical and especially mental, before they are able to accept their disability and make the most of what is left to them. They may feel considerable bitterness and resentment at what has befallen them. It is often better for such persons to receive help in a residential rehabilitation centre where the course aims at re-establishing self-confidence in the performance of daily activities and in mobility. As well as learning to read and write Braille, those who are young enough will be given vocational training. Where it is not possible for a newly blinded person to be resident at a rehabilitation course considerable help is available from the staff of the local authority social services departments. St Dunstan's provides help for blind people who have served in the armed forces and also for firemen and policemen blinded on duty.

Most blind people of working age are employed on equal terms with sighted people in offices and industry. Help is available through the employment service agency to find a suitable job and to provide 'on-the-job' training to ensure that the blind employee can do his work safely and effectively. For some blind adults sheltered employment is necessary and is provided either in workshops for the blind or in home-workers schemes administered by local authorities or voluntary agencies.

Piano tuning has become a traditional occupation for blind people and is one which offers scope for those who wish to be self-employed. The RNIB provides specialist placement services for people wishing to be employed in commercial and professional fields and for those who wish to return to the occupation they followed before losing their sight.

When elderly people become newly blind special problems arise. They often find it easier to learn Moon type rather than Braille. Rather than admit them to a home for the blind, special encouragement and help should be given to enable them to continue living in their own homes for as long as possible. Much reassurance and support will be needed for such people from their families, neighbours and the social services department. The increased number of elderly and infirm blind people in recent years has led to the provision of purpose-built special accommodation for them. Some blind people are cared for in the homes for the elderly provided by the local authority social services department.

SERVICES FOR THE BLIND

Reading materials, including newspapers, weekly and monthly periodicals and a special edition of the *Radio Times*, are obtainable in Braille or Moon type. Books are available either for purchase or on loan and this service includes textbooks. For those with poor sight books with large print may be obtained from public libraries.

Light-weight magnetic tape cassettes, known as 'talking books', on a wide range of subjects are also available and are played on a special playback machine. Portable VHF radios are provided through the British Wireless for the Blind Fund. Games and appliances such as watches have been specially designed for the needs of the blind. There are also certain aids in the home, for instance a Braille temperature control can be fitted to gas stoves.

Travel concessions are provided in some areas and under certain circumstances British Rail allows a blind person and a guide to travel for the price of one adult fare.

The Guide Dogs for the Blind Association provides and trains special dogs to guide the blind. The selection and training of the dogs and the blind person is lengthy and therefore only a small number of carefully chosen people can benefit by this service.

Holiday homes and hostels specially designed for the safety of blind people also exist. Many are run by voluntary bodies with the running cost supplied by the local authority.

Many people who lose their sight are very concerned about their financial position. There are a wide range of benefits available from the Department of Health and Social Security, e.g. disablement benefit, attendance allowance. If these are not sufficient to meet the needs of the blind person or his family, supplementary benefit at a higher rate is payable to registered blind people. In addition financial assistance may be available from voluntary agencies. Extra income tax relief is allowed.

The nurse who works amongst people with diseases of the eye must be aware of how she can help patients who are already blind. For those who have recently become blind, and their relatives, the nurse should be able to give some indication of the services available as described briefly above, but should refer them to the medical social worker for detailed information.

When a blind person is received into a ward he may be temporarily confused because his surroundings are unfamiliar; the nurse has a considerable role to play in helping the patient adapt and settle down. The disability of blindness inevitably imposes limitations on the blind person, but these vary from one individual to another and it is important for the nurse to find out the potential of each person and enable him to live as normally as possible.

A blind person newly admitted to a ward must be allowed to familiarize himself with his surroundings by being shown round and allowed to feel the position of the furniture until he is competent to manage by himself under the overall supervision of the nursing staff. The newly blind may feel safe only in a very restricted sphere and will need help from the nurse whenever he has to move somewhere new. In general doors should be kept shut and if it is necessary to move the position of furniture for any reason it is essential to warn the patient of the change. When leading a blind person it should be borne in mind that he will often prefer to take the nurse's arm rather than allow her to take his.

When talking to a patient who is blind it is helpful to tell him who you are and your status in the ward, and in other small ways, such as letting him know you are about ot leave, make sure he understands what is going on around him. If several patients are together the nurse can touch the arm of the patient to whom she is speaking.

There are many ways in which a nurse, by using her imagination and trying to put herself into the place of the blind patient can help him to feel more secure during his stay in the hospital ward.

Glossary

Abscise	To cut away
Accommodation	The power of the lens to become more convex and so allow near objects to be focussed
Amblyopia	Reduced vision in an eye of normal appearance
Aphakic	Eye from which the lens has been removed
Astigmatism	Irregularity of the corneal or lens surface
Aqueous humour	A watery fluid which is constantly secreted by the ciliary body, circulates in the anterior chamber and drains away at the angle between the cornea and the outer edge of the iris
Blepharitis	Inflammation of the lid margins
Blepharospasm	Spasm of the eyelids
Canthus	The angles formed by the junction of the lids, inner and outer
Cataract	Opacity of the lens
Cartella shield	Protective eye shield
Caruncle	The normal nodular elevation of the inner canthus of the eye

Chemosis	Oedema of the conjunctiva
Choroid	The vascular lining of the eyeball
Ciliary body	The part of the uveal tract between iris and choroid which contains the muscles of accommodation and secretes aqueous
Cilium	Eyelash
Commotio retinae	Oedema of the retina after ocular contusion
Cycloplegia	Paralysis of the ciliary muscle
Dacryocystitis	Inflammation of the lacrimal sac
Diplopia	Double vision
Discission	Operation for soft cataract when the anterior lens capsule is ruptured to allow the lens substance to be absorbed, or removed
Distichiasis	Double row of eyelashes
Ectropion	Eversion of the eyelid
Emmetropia	Normal sight
Endemic	A disease prevalent in a particular locality
Endogenous	Coming from within
Entropion	Abnormal inward displacement of the lid margin towards the eye
Enucleation	Surgical removal of the entire eye including the sclera
Epicanthus	A vertical fold of skin at the inner canthus of the eye
Epidemic	A disease attacking a large number of people at the same time
Epilation	Removal of eye lashes
Epiphora	Overflow of tears due to inadequate drainage
Evisceration	Removal of the eye excluding the sclera
Exenteration of orbit	Removal of all the soft tissues in the orbit
Exophthalmus	Prominence of the eyeball, usually both eyes are affected

Fornix	The point at which the bulbar conjunctiva is reflected on to the eyelid to meet the palpebral conjunctiva and a loose pouch is formed
Fundus	The portion of the retina which can be seen with an ophthalmoscope
Glaucoma	Raised intraocular pressure
Hordeolum	External stye; inflammation of the sebaceous glands of the eyelashes
Hypermetropia	Long sight
Hyphaema	Blood in the anterior chamber
Hypopyon	Pus in the anterior chamber
Iridectomy	Removal of part of the iris
Iridocyclitis	Inflammation of the iris and the ciliary body
Iridodialysis	Tearing of the iris from the ciliary body
Iris	The coloured part of the eye
Ischaemia	Lack of blood to a part
Keratitis	Inflammation of the cornea
Keratoplasty	Corneal grafting (transplantation)
Lacrimation	Excessive production of tears
Limbus	Junction of the cornea with the sclera
Macula lutea	Area of most acute vision on the retina
Meibomian cyst	Internal hordeolum of the meibomian gland near to the lid margin
Meibomian glands	Sebaceous glands of the eyelids
Miotic	An agent which constricts the pupil
Mydriatic	An agent which dilates the pupil
Myopia	Short sight
Needling	Capsulotomy: the capsule of the lens is torn with a special needle
Nematode	A genus of worms, including the round worm and the thread worm
Nystagmus	Rhythmic involuntary oscillation of the eye

Onchocerciasis	A filariasis caused by *Onchocerca volvulus*
Ophthalmia neonatorum	Ophthalmia of the newborn
Optic cup	Central depression in the optic disc
Ora serrata	Anterior boundary of the retina
Panophthalmitis	Generalized infection of the eye
Paracentesis	Tapping of the anterior chamber
Photophobia	Sensitivity to light
Phthisis bulbi	Soft atrophic destruction of the eye
Presbyopia	Reduced power of accommodation due to advancing age
Proptosis	Prominence of the eyeball and lids
Pupil	Central opening encircled by the iris
Recession	Muscle cut from insertion and reattached posteriorly
Refraction	The testing of vision
Resection	Removal of a section of muscle
Retina	Light sensitive layer of the eye
Rhodopsin	Visual purple of the rods
Sarcoidosis	A rare disease in some ways similar to tuberculosis which may affect the eye
Schlemm, canal of	Aqueous drainage channel encircling the periphery of the anterior chamber
Sclera	Tough white outer layer of the eye
Scotoma	A defect in the field of vision
Stenosis	Narrowing or contracting of a channel or opening
Strabismus	Squint
Symblepharon	Adhesion of the lid to the eyeball
Synechia	Adhesion of the iris to the lens behind or to the cornea in front
Tarsorrhaphy	Suturing together of the lid margins, in total or part
Tenon's capsule	Sheath of connective tissue encircling the eyeball and orbit

Trabecula	Meshwork in the anterior chamber through which the aqueous flows to leave the eye
Trichiasis	Lashes that turn against the cornea
Trochlea	Fibrous pulley of the superior oblique muscle
Uveitis	Inflammation of the pigmented layer of the eye comprising the iris, ciliary body and choroid
Vitreous humour	A gelatinous, transparent substance varying in density enclosed in a hyaline membrane lying posterior to the lens
Zonule	Suspensory ligament which suspends the lens

Index

accommodation, 35
acetazolamide, 85, 99
albinism, 100
amblyopia, 136
anti-histamine drops, 31
anti-inflammatory drugs, 30
antimicrobials, 30
aqueous humour, 79
arcus senilis, 104
artery
    facial, 118
    ophthalmic, 118
    palpebral, 118
artificial eye, 168
    fitting, 168
    removal, 170
astigmatism, 39

bacterial endocarditis, 67
Bell's phenomenon, 147
Blaskovic's operation, 149
blepharitis, 149
blepharospasm, 107
blind services, 175
    see also schooling
blindness
    in adults, 173
    in children, 172
    colour, 67

Bowman's membrane, 104
Braille, 175
buphthalmos, see glaucoma,
        congenital
Burkitt's lymphoma, 162
    treatment, 163

canal of Schlemm, 79
canthus, 147
carbonic anhydrase inhibitor, 85
caruncle, 118
cataract, 40
    complicated, 56
    congenital and developmental,
        51
        causes, 51
        operation, 52
        postoperative care, 53
        preoperative care, 52
    diabetic, 54
    operation, 44–7
    senile, 40
    traumatic, 54
'cat's eye reflex', 75
cavernous sinus thrombosis, 143
central retinal arterial
        thrombosis, 67
central retinal vein
        thrombosis, 66

chalazion, *see* meibomian cyst
chemical burns, 123
chemosis, 76
chickenpox, 154
choroid, 100
choroiditis, 102
chymotrypsin, 45
ciliary body, 100
ciliary injection, 100
ciliary muscles, 100
ciliary processes, 100
cobalt therapy in
        retinoblastoma, 75
collagen diseases, 101
colour blindness, 67
commotio retinae, 69
concretions, 162
contact lenses, 56
  removal, 57, 59
conjunctiva, 118
  chemical burns, 123
conjunctival sac, 146
conjunctival swab, 19
conjunctivitis, 119
  acute infective, 120
  allergic, 123
  viral, 122
cornea, 104
  foreign bodies, 113
  grafting, *see* keratoplasty
  injury, 113
  ulceration, 107
corneoscleral lens, 56
counselling, genetic, 76
cranial nerves, 135
cryotherapy, 108, 73
cyclodialysis, 92
cyclodiathermy, 92
cyclophosphamide, 163
cycloplegics, 28

dacryocystectomy, 131
dacryocystitis, 130
dacryocystography, 129

dacryocystorrhinostomy, 131
dark—light adaptation, 63
dendritic ulcer, 107
dermatitis, allergic, 153
Descemet's membrane, 104
diabetes mellitus, 54, 101
Diamox, *see* acetazolamide
diethylcarbamizine, 161
digital palpation, 81
diplopia, 135
Disablement Resettlement Officer,
    74
discission, 52
distant vision, estimation, 10
distichiasis, 147
donor eyes, 110
Down's syndrome, 148
drainage angle, 79
drops
  classification, 27.
  instillation, 13, 14
  reaction, 28, 32
  types
    adrenaline, 91
    antazoline, 31
    anti-histamine, 31
    atropine, 28
    Bengal rose, 31
    chloramphenicol, 30
    cocaine, 31
    cyclopentolate, 28
    dyflos, 30
    ecothiopate, 30
    eserine, *see* physostigmine
    fluorescein, 31, 106
    homatropine, 28
    hypomellose, 31
    idoxuridine, 30
    lachesine, 28
    methylcellulose, 31
    neomycin, 30
    paroleine, 144
    phenylephrine, 28
    physostigmine, 28, 29
    pilocarpine, 29, 91

drops (*continued*)
    types (*continued*)
        steroids, 30
        sulphacetamide, 122
ducts
    lacrimal, 130
    nasolacrimal, 128

eclipse, 68
ectropion, 153
electrolysis, 147
electro-oculogram, 66
electroradiogram, 66
emmetropia, 36
endocarditis, bacterial, 67
entropion, 153
enucleation, 166
    for retinoblastoma, 75
    postoperative care, 167
    preoperative care, 167
epicanthus, 136, 148
epilation, 22
epilation forceps, 22
epiphora, 129, 152
episcleral tissue, 117
episcleritis, 117
eserine, *see* physostigmine
E test, 11
ethmoidal sinus, 141
ethmoiditis, 141
Everbusch's operation, 149
eversion of lid, 16
evisceration, 170
examination of eye, 41
exenteration, 170
exophthalmic goitre, 144
exophthalmos, 144
extraocular muscles, 133
eye banks, 110
eyebrows, 156
eyedrops, *see* drops
eyelashes, 22, 146
eyelids, 145–7
    eversion, 16

eyelids (*continued*)
    infections, 149
    muscles, 148
    oedema, 142
    tumours, 155

facial nerve paralysis, 108
Fisher's dish, 17
filarial infections, 160
focussing, 38
foreign bodies
    corneal, 113
    intraocular, 114
    subtarsal, 148

genetic counselling, 76
glands
    meibomian, 146
    of Moll, 147
    of Zeis, 147
glass shell, 168
glasses, smoked, 68
glaucoma, 82
    absolute, 92
    closed-angle, 82
        postoperative care, 87
        preoperative care, 86
        treatment, 84
    congenital, 93
        operation, 94
        postoperative care, 94
        preoperative care, 93
    open-angle, 87
        treatment, 91
    secondary, 92
    steroid, 92
    thrombotic, 93
grafts
    conjunctival, 125
    corneal, 109
glycerol, 86
gonioscopic mirror, 81

herpetic ulceration, 107
herpes zoster ophthalmicus, 154
    treatment, 155
hordeolum
    external, 150
    internal, *see* meibomian cyst
hot spoon bathing, 20
Human Tissue Act, 110
hyaloid canal, 34
hyaloid fossa, 33
hypermetropia, 39
hyphaema, 49, 98
    traumatic, 69
hypopyon, 101

injury
    corneal, 113
    of iris, 98
    of lens, 54
instillation
    of drops, 13, 14
    of ointment, 15
intraocular foreign bodies, 114
    postoperative care, 115
    preoperative care, 115
intraocular lenses, 55
intraocular pressure, 80
    measurement, 81
    rise, 82
iridocyclitis, 100
iridodialysis, 97
iris
    bombé, 101
    injury, 98
        complications, 98
        treatment, 99
    muscles, 97
    pigment, 97
    prolapse, 64
iritis, *see* iridocyclitis
irradiation, 108
irrigation of eye, 17

Jaeger's test type, 12

keratic precipitates, 101, 102
keratitis, 105
    disciform, 109
    exposure, 108
    interstitial, 109
    non-ulcerative, 109
    striate, 49
    symptoms, 106
    ulcerative, 107
keratoconjunctivitis
    chronic, 158
    epidemic, 159
keratomalacia, 163
keratoplasty, 109
    lamellar, 110
    operation, 111
    penetrating, 110
    postoperative care, 112
    preoperative care, 111

lachesine, 28
lacrimal ducts
    acquired obstruction, 130
    congenital obstruction, 130
lacrimal gland, 127
lacrimal passages
    syringing, 23
    trauma, 132
lacrimal sac, 128
    syringing, 23
lacrimal syringe, 24
lacrimation, 129
laser beam, 73
lashes, 146
    cutting, 22
    epilation, 22
lens, 33—5
    capsule, 33
lens extraction
    extracapsular, 44
    intracapsular, 45

lens extraction (*continued*)
　intracapsular (*continued*)
　　first dressing, 48
　　operation, 44
　　postoperative care, 47
　　postoperative complications, 51
　　preoperative care, 42
lenses, contact, 56
　corneoscleral, 56
　haptic, 56
　microcorneal, 56
　soft, 56
leprosy, 164
levator palpabrae, 148
leucoma, 106
light coagulation therapy, 75
light coagulator, 73
limbus, 104
lime burns, 123
Loa loa, 161
local anaesthetics, 31
long sight (hypermetropia), 39
lymphoma of orbit, 162
lysozyme, 127

macula lutea, 61, 66
Maddox heater, 21, 22
malnutrition, 163
mannitol, 86
meibomian cyst, 150
meibomian glands, 146, 150
melanoma of iris, 103
methotrexate, 163
microcorneal lenses, 56
miotics, 29
Moon type, 174
Mooren's ulcer, 108
mucocele, 130
muscles
　ciliary, 100
　eyelid, 148
　extraocular, 133
　iris, 97

muscles (*continued*)
　oblique, 134
　recti, 133
mydriatic test, 91
mydriasis, traumatic, 99
mydriatics, 27
Mydricaine, 25, 28
myopia, 37
　retinal separation in, 69

nasolacrimal duct, 128
near vision, 35
nebula, 106
needling, 45
Nettleship's dilator, 23
nystagmus, 100

occlusion, 136
oedema of lids, 142
onchocerciasis, 160
ophthalmia neonatorum, 121, 161
ophthalmoscope, 65
optic chiasma, 64
optic cup, 67
optic disc, 63
　cupping, 87
optic foramen, 140
optic nerve, 63
orbit, 140
　fractures, 145
　tumours, 145
　see also Burkitt's lymphoma
orbital cellulitis, 142
orthoptic exercises, 137
orthoptist, 136
out-patient clinics, 9

palpation, digital, 81
panophthalmitis, 142
paracentesis of anterior chamber, 67
perimeter, 88

phakoemulsification, 47
phasing, *see* tonometry
photocoagulation, 73
photophobia, 106, 119
phthisis bulbi, 122
pigment epithelium of retina, 69
pinguecula, 126
postoperative care, general
  principles, 4–6, 7, 8
  see also specific disorders
presbyopia, 39
pressure, intraocular, 80
procaine, 31
proptosis, 144
protective goggles, 113
pterygium, 126
ptosis, 148
puncta, 24, 128
pupillary block, 83

recession, 138
recti muscles, 133
refraction
  errors, 36–9
  of light, 36
Reiter's syndrome, 122
resection, 138
retina, 61
  artery, 67
  contusion, 69
  degeneration, 66
  detachment, *see* retina,
    separation
  separation, 69–71
    operations, 73
    ophthalmic examin-
      ation, 66
    postoperative care, 74
    preoperative care, 71
    primary, 69
    secondary, 69
  tear, 70
  vein, 66
retinitis pigmentosa, 67

retinoblastoma, 75
  preoperative care, 75
  postoperative care, 76
river blindness, *see* onchocerciasis
rhodopsin, 62
rodding, 24, 125
rodent ulcer, 155
rods and cones, 61
Royal National Institute for the
  Blind, 111, 172
rubella, 51

sarcoidosis, 102
Schlemm, canal of, 79, 117
schooling for the blind, 172, 173
sclera, 116
scleritis, 117
scotoma, 88
shell, glass, 168
Sheridan test, 12
short sight (myopia), 37
sight
  long, 39
  normal, 35
  short, 37
  see also vision
silicone
  plombs, 73
  rod, 73
sinuses, nasal, 141
Sjögren's disease, 127
slit-lamp, 35
smallpox, 164
Snellen's test type, 10
soft lenses, 56
solar retinopathy, 68
squint, *see* strabismus
staphyloma, 117
strabismus, 135
  correction, 138
  operations, 138
  postoperative care, 138
  preoperative care, 138
  treatment, 136

streptococcal infections, 101
stye, *see* hordeolum, external
subconjunctival haemorrhage, 123
subconjunctival injection, 25
    drugs by, 25, 28
sulphones, 164
suspensory ligament, 34
symblepharon, 124, 125, 158
sympathetic ophthalmia, 116
synechia, 53, 101

tarsal plate, 16, 146
tarsorrhaphy, 108, 144
tears, composition of, 127
Tenon's capsule, 117
tests
    dark room, 89
    fluorescein, 129
    mydriatic, 91
    Schirmer's, 128
    water drinking, 89
thrombosis
    cevernous sinus, 143
    central retinal arterial, 67
    central retinal vein, 66
thyrotoxic exophthalmos, 144
tonographic measurement, 81
tonometer, 81
tonometry, 81
toxoplasmosis, 102
trabecula, 79
trabeculectomy, 92
trachoma, 158
trichiasis, 149
trigeminal nerve, 154
tuberculosis, 102

ulceration
    corneal, 107
    dendritic, 107
    herpetic, 107
    limbus, 56

undine, 17
uveal tract, 96
    tumours, 100
uveitis, 100
    causes, 101
    granulomatous, 102
    posterior, 102
    treatment, 101

vision
    binocular, 135
    colour, 62
    distant, 10
        estimation, 10
    daylight, 62
    near, 35
    see also sight
visual acuity, 9
visual fields
    charting, 88
    defects, 88
visual pathway, 63
visual purple, 61
vitamin A, 62
    deficiency, 163
vitamin B deficiency, 163
vitreous, 78
    body, 78
    loss, 79
    opacities, 79
    replacement, 79

xerophthalmia, 163

yellow spot, 61

zonule, 34